THE HISTORY OF NURSING IN NORTH CAROLINA

D1563676

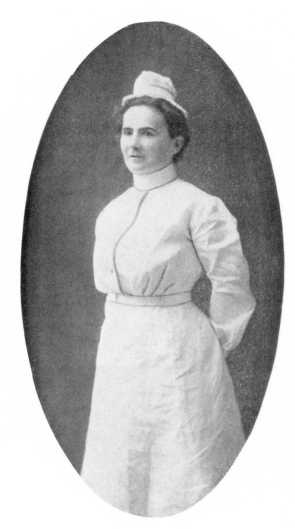

Mary Lewis Wyche

THE HISTORY OF
NURSING
IN NORTH CAROLINA

BY
MARY LEWIS WYCHE

EDITED BY
EDNA L. HEINZERLING

CHAPEL HILL

THE UNIVERSITY OF NORTH CAROLINA PRESS

TO

ALL THOSE NURSES IN

NORTH CAROLINA

WHO MADE

THIS HISTORY POSSIBLE

THE NURSE

Tall daughter of an ancient race, she stands
Benign and beautiful and strong and wise.
The world, like a tired child beneath her hands
Sleeps and is healed.

So often her grave eyes have looked on pain and death,
That by her will
The terrors of the night are held at bay—
Under her touch our quivering nerves are still
And all the thirsty torment of the day
Is bearable because her strength is near.

Her heart with service as its chosen star
Helps us to overcome our sickly fear
And where she is, hope and compassion are;
Thus excellently power and pity blend
In Healer, Mother, Comforter and Friend.

—Oriana Atkinson, New York Times, 1935

FOREWORD

MARY LEWIS WYCHE, of Raleigh, first conceived the idea of publishing an historical account of nursing in North Carolina. She collected the data and wrote part of the history through the years preceding 1930. When her labor of love was interrupted by ill health and eventually by death, the manuscript was purchased by the North Carolina Board of Nurse Examiners, with the agreement that the book should be completed and published under her name.

Members of the North Carolina State Nurses' Association, anxious to preserve their history, made arrangements through a committee appointed by the president of the association to have the history compiled and completed by Edna L. Heinzerling. The work has been financed by funds secured from the Federal government through the Works Progress Administration and the North Carolina State Nurses' Association.

From histories, from old library records, and from personal interviews with a score of veteran nurses in the State, the information found in this volume was compiled. The whole story of nursing in North Carolina is a mosaic made up of many pieces representing the individual ministry of a host of faithful nurses to suffering humanity.

The committee is grateful to Mary Hunter for research work; to Lula West for her untiring efforts in obtaining correct data, making revisions, and reading the manuscript;

and to Dr. Wingate M. Johnson, for reading and correcting the manuscript.

HETTIE REINHARDT, *chairman*
BESSIE M. CHAPMAN
MRS. DOROTHY CONYERS
BIRDIE DUNN
MRS. EMILY JENKINS PICKARD
JOSEPHINE KERR
BLANCHE STAFFORD

INTRODUCTION

MARY LEWIS WYCHE

Mary Lewis Wyche was born February 26, 1858, near Henderson. She was the daughter of Benjamin and Sara Hunter Wyche. Her life of dauntless courage, sincerity, and integrity is characteristic of her fine ancestry and of the family environment in which she was reared. It is a beautiful story of love for her younger brothers and sisters and for all humanity.

Miss Wyche, with a younger sister, was graduated from Henderson College in June, 1889. While a student there she taught in the primary department of the school. Soon after leaving college she went to Chapel Hill to make a home for her younger brothers who were preparing to enter the University of North Carolina. At different times while there she kept boarders and taught as a means of livelihood. These early struggles, perhaps, and her ardent belief in the education of youth caused her later to aid, with small loans, several young students to enter college.

When her brothers no longer needed assistance, Miss Wyche directed her thoughts to her own life work. She first thought of preparing for a medical career, but later she decided to enter the nursing profession. This was practically a new field for women of the higher type. After graduating from the Philadelphia General Hospital in 1894 at the age of thirty-six, she returned to North Carolina to give hundreds of young women of her native state the value of her wise counsel during the period of organization.

Under her capable supervision Rex Hospital Training School for nurses was organized in Raleigh in October, 1894, with five student nurses in the first class, four of whom graduated. For three years she remained as superintendent of nurses, resigning in 1898 to do private duty nursing in Raleigh. A year later she accepted the position of charge nurse of the infirmary of State Normal and Industrial College, Greensboro. In 1901 she returned to Raleigh and was engaged in private duty nursing one year.

Miss Wyche realized the necessity of state organization for nurses if North Carolina were to become a leader in the profession. Her first important public work was the organization of the Raleigh Nurses' Association in 1901, a forerunner of the North Carolina State Nurses' Association. Recognizing the fact that further study was also necessary for her own advancement, she went to Philadelphia later in 1901 to spend a year in the study of dietetics and massage.

Upon her return to North Carolina she accepted the position of superintendent of nurses at Watts Hospital, Durham, remaining there from 1903 to 1913. Under her wise direction the hospital and school made splendid progress. A large addition was built to the hospital during her administration.

In 1902 Mary Lewis Wyche, with fourteen other nurses, organized the North Carolina State Nurses' Association. She served as its president six years. Through her untiring efforts a law for compulsory registration of graduate nurses was passed in 1903. North Carolina was the first state in the Union to get this law passed. Like other pioneer nurses she took a prominent part in all nursing activities and held offices of importance in the early days. She was the first chairman of the legislative committee for state registration and also secretary-treasurer of the first Board of Examiners for Trained Nurses, serving six years in the latter capacity.

Miss Wyche was very much interested in a home for tubercular nurses. When Birdie Dunn presented the idea for such a home to the State Nurses' Association she was assisted by Miss Wyche in securing funds to start the home. Later Miss Wyche gave much of her time to the work of planning and opening this home, which bore the name of Dunnwyche. She went back to hospital work in 1915 and became superintendent of Sarah Elizabeth Hospital in Henderson, remaining there two years.

The movement to establish a prenursing course at the North Carolina College for Women at Greensboro was led by this remarkable woman, and she was the first to ask that a school of nursing be established in connection with Duke University at Durham.

After leaving Sarah Elizabeth Hospital in 1917, Miss Wyche engaged in private duty nursing in Greensboro and Raleigh until 1925, when she retired from active service and began the work of compiling a history of nursing in North Carolina.

At a banquet of the North Carolina State Nurses' Association in Raleigh in 1932, she was presented a bar pin and a card bearing a simple inscription of grateful recognition of her work. This pin was highly prized and often worn.

Miss Wyche was honorary president of the North Carolina State Nurses' Association and remained in this office until her death, August 22, 1936. Her last years were spent in her childhood home, "Wychewood." Many of the friends and neighbors of her early years had moved from the community but she was grateful for visits from faithful friends who came from various sections of the state to comfort and cheer her in her last days.

The clear vision and wise counsel of Mary Lewis Wyche had a far-reaching effect on the young women who had their training under her supervision. Her sincerity and devotion to the cause of nursing can never be estimated. In every phase of her versatile life as student, teacher, nurse, hospital superintendent, and organizer, the spirit of the crusader prevailed.

CONTENTS

PAGE

FOREWORD vii

INTRODUCTION ix

I. EARLY NURSING IN NORTH CAROLINA 3

II. MILITARY NURSING 9

III. HOSPITALS AND SCHOOLS FOR NURSES 26

IV. PIONEER NURSES AND LEADERS 51

V. NURSING ORGANIZATIONS 66

VI. STATE EDUCATIONAL DIRECTORS 90

VII. LEGISLATION AND REGISTRATION FOR NURSES 95

VIII. DUNNWYCHE AND THE NURSES' RELIEF FUND 111

IX. PUBLIC HEALTH NURSING 116

X. THE ESTABLISHMENT OF NEGRO HOSPITALS AND THE
PROGRESS OF NEGRO NURSES 126

IN MEMORIAM 132

APPENDICES 135

BIBLIOGRAPHY 145

INDEX 147

ILLUSTRATIONS

Mary Lewis Wyche.............................*Frontispiece*

Facing page

Etta Mae Perkins... 24
Annie Dade Reveley....................................... 24
Bessie Mordecai 25
Rosa G. Hill... 25
Rex Hospital, Raleigh, 1894.............................. 34
Rex Hospital, Raleigh, 1937.............................. 34
Twin-City Hospital, Winston-Salem, 1895.................. 35
City Memorial Hospital, Winston-Salem, 1938.............. 35
Highsmith Hospital, Fayetteville......................... 42
Watts Hospital, Durham................................... 42
Dr. Henry F. Long's Hospital, Statesville................ 43
James Walker Memorial Hospital, Wilmington............... 43
St. Peter's Hospital, Charlotte.......................... 48
Asheville Mission Hospital............................... 48
State Hospital for the Insane, Raleigh................... 49
Adeline Orr 54
Mollie Spach 54
Jane Christmas Yancey.................................... 55
Mary Rose Batterham...................................... 55
Mary Lewis Wyche... 66
Constance E. Pfohl....................................... 66
Cleone E. Hobbs.. 66
L. Eugenia Henderson..................................... 66
Blanche Stafford 67
Dorothy Conyers 67
Pearl Weaver 67
Columbia Munds 67
Mary P. Laxton... 74
Miss E. A. Kelley.. 74
Hettie Reinhardt 74
Ruth Council 74
Mrs. Marion H. Laurance.................................. 75
Mrs. E. Irby Long.. 75
First Public Health Nurses............................... 75
Page from Secretary-Treasurer's Book..................... 110
Dunnwyche 111

THE HISTORY OF
NURSING
IN
NORTH CAROLINA

THE

FLORENCE NIGHTINGALE

PLEDGE

I solemnly pledge myself before God and in the presence of this assembly to pass my life in purity and to practice my profession faithfully. I will abstain from whatever is deleterious or mischievous and will not take or knowingly administer any harmful drug. I will do all in my power to elevate the standard of my profession and will hold in confidence all personal matters committed to my keeping, and all family affairs coming to my knowledge in the practice of my calling. With loyalty will I endeavor to aid the physician in his work, and devote myself to the welfare of those committed to my care.

CHAPTER I

EARLY NURSING IN NORTH CAROLINA

THE HISTORY of nursing in North Carolina has been made in the last three decades of the twentieth century. The early records deal more with the health laws which were made to safeguard the welfare of the people than with medicine and nursing as we have it today.

Apparently the first public care of the sick in the Colony of Carolina of which there is any record was given to a woman in the Precinct of Chowan in 1703. From the Vestry Book of St. Paul's Parish at Edenton under date of "April ye 4th, 1703," the following account is found:

"Information being made by Capt^t Thomas Blount that Elinor Adams by of Infirmity and Indigence is in great Danger of being lost for want of Assistance.

"The Same being taken into Consideration—Ordered that Captt. Thomas Blount treat with Doc^r Godfrey Spruill in order to her Cure and that Doctor Godfrey Spruill be paid for his physick and Care by the Church Wardens five pounds, and Capt. Thomas Blount is requested by Vestry to endeavour to oblige the Said Elenor to Serve the Doctor for the use of his House and nursing."[1]

The early colonists considered vital statistics so important that they had laws which imposed a penalty if these records were not kept. A provision of the Fundamental Constitu-

[1] *Colonial Records,* I, 569.

tion stated that the age of everyone born in Carolina should be reckoned from the day that the birth was entered in the registry and not before. Failure to report births and deaths within two months resulted in a penalty of five shillings a week. It is literally true that no native Carolinian was considered anybody unless his birth was on record.[2]

Laws passed in 1738 relative to contagious diseases were forerunners of our modern quarantine laws. The attention of the authorities was called to smallpox on board a shipload of Negroes from South Carolina and expulsion of the ship was ordered by the Council of State. The master of the ship was ordered to keep himself and the patients apart and to take the ship two miles up the Black River for three weeks.[3]

The following advertisement and recommendation of a trained midwife in North Carolina was found among very old papers:

"Mid-wife Advertisement

"Agnes Mackinley, midwife from Glasgow

"Respectfully offers her services to the Ladies of Wilmington and its vicinity, and begs leave to solicit their favors in the line of her business. She has been in this town since July last, but indisposition precluded her making a tender of her services to the public till now.

"She will likewise attend Ladies in Fayetteville if sent for.

"As the encouragement she hopes for must depend in a great degree on her being properly qualified for the above business, and as a proof thereof, she subjoins the following certificate:

"These are to certify that Mrs. Agnes Mackinley has regularly attended my Course of Lectures in Midwifery, for one session of the College, and has undergone all the usual Examinations with approbation; and further, that the said Mrs.

[2] *Ibid.*, II, 877.   [3] *Ibid.*, IV, 333-34.

Agnes Mackinley has pursued the knowledge and practice
of Midwifery under my directions at the Lying-in-Hospital,
where she had opportunities assisting at a variety of Labour's.

"In testimoney whereof, this certificate is subscribed to
me, March 8, 1789. JAMES TOWERS, A. O. P.

59"[4]

With very few physicians available and no organized
nursing, except that of the Moravians, the care of the sick
was of necessity the responsibility of each household. From
authentic records which have been preserved by the Moravians, a few instances can be cited which show that they
had very good nursing service for their time. It will be re-
called that they entered the State through the Albemarle
section from Pennsylvania in 1752, and had to travel over a
pathless forest to reach Wachovia, now Forsyth County.
They met with many disasters and were the victims of various types of diseases. The journey was beset with hardships, including a number of cases of fever, probably malaria
contracted at Edenton. Bishop Spangenberg, describing in
his diary these cases of chills and fever, reports they were all
ill, except "Br. Joseph Müller" who was their "Faithful and
unwearying nurse."[5] The patients were treated by sweating
produced by the use of a root found in the Albemarle section. This was used presumably to allay the high fever.

Among the party of eleven unmarried men who came
to Wachovia in 1753 was a surgeon, Dr. Hans Martin Kalberlahn, who served not only the Moravians, but the surrounding county. He stands out in history because of his
knowledge of surgery and disease. His wise counsel was
eagerly sought by people far and near; patients were brought
a hundred miles and more to consult him.[6] On one occasion

[4] Hall's *Wilmington Gazette*, March 8, 1798.
[5] Adelaide L. Fries (ed.), *Records of the Moravians in North Carolina*, I, 43.
[6] *Ibid.*, pp. 105, 173.

he operated on a man who had been struck on the head with an axe. He removed a piece of bone from the skull. The patient's mind had become affected by the accident, so Dr. Kalberlahn kept him under observation several days.[7] Other services performed by him were treatment of deafness,[8] dental work, and taking care of victims of accidents incident to the work of building.

Amusing stories are told of the remuneration which was offered Dr. Kalberlahn for his services. From one patient he received two cows valued at fifty shillings each; from another, a cow and calf, and from still another the promise of two bushels of corn. Among the brethren's possessions were a few books and Dr. Kalberlahn borrowed them for his patients or had someone read to them to help pass the tedious hours of illness.[9]

As the Moravians had to depend on their own resources for medicine, one of the first plantings was a "medical garden." A plan of one of these gardens may be seen in the Wachovia Land Office.[10] An interesting list of the medical herbs gathered is recorded. A laboratory and drug store was established by the early settlers.[11]

Five years after Dr. Kalberlahn arrived in North Carolina, he decided to return to Pennsylvania for a visit. Before leaving, he taught several of the brethren to "let blood" and gave them other instructions in medicine.

When he returned to Carolina in 1759 with his bride, who was a great help to him in caring for the sick, he found that the Indians had been at war with each other and that many of the refugees were either wounded or ill from exposure. At Bethabara an epidemic of typhus fever raged for five or six months. Dr. Kalberlahn was deeply grieved because he could not do more for his brethren and friends.

[7] *Ibid.*, p. 124.
[8] *Ibid.*, p. 171.   [9] *Ibid.*, p. 133 ff.
[10] John Henry Clewell, *History of Wachovia in North Carolina*, p. 24.
[11] *Ibid.*, p. 60.

Many died and it is probable that the effect of this epidemic caused his own death on July 28, 1759.

In 1835 the United States Medical Society placed a new stone on Dr. Kalberlahn's grave in the Oldtown Graveyard at Bethabara. An additional stone placed just below the gravestone bears this inscription: "First Doctor of Wachovia."

The Moravians had a system of providing what they called a "sick-room" for the brethren. It was set up whenever or wherever needed and certain brethren were appointed to do the nursing. In the Wachovia Historical Society building, Winston-Salem, there may be seen in a glass case a small card containing the names of sixteen men. Opposite the names are days of the week, and underneath the following is written: "Sick nurses appointed for the year 1810, Moravian Congregation, Salem, N. C."

To indicate the need of help in a distant locality, the brethren rang bells, blew trumpets, or fired guns. Answering one of the calls they found a woman and her four children fleeing from the Indians.[12] On another occasion a white man was rescued with an arrow protruding from his back. He received successful treatment from Dr. Jacob Bonn who had come to Salem to take the place of Dr. Kalberlahn.[13]

Salem had a remarkably modern health department as early as 1772. There was a community doctor, an appointed midwife, and nurses. The neighbors were frequently called upon to nurse each other and no distance was too great for them to go and give several hours' service regardless of home cares and other duties. Dr. Bonn gave these women instructions in the art of nursing.

In the light of their refusal to bear arms because of religious scruples, the Moravians' care of the sick and wounded who were brought to Salem during the Revolutionary War

[12] Fries, *op. cit.*, I, 134.   [13] Clewell, *op. cit.*, p. 48.

seems all the more commendable. Many of these disabled soldiers remained several months and received tender nursing and the most skillful surgical care. In fact, Dr. Bonn is said to have effected some marvelous results in the case of many severely wounded soldiers.

About this time Salem experienced a smallpox epidemic. Dr. Bonn hesitated to inoculate against the disease because of the sick and wounded, but he used every precaution to keep the soldiers from contracting it.[14]

Soon after the Revolutionary War the unmarried sisters built a large house similar to the one occupied by the brethren. Here they had their "sick-rooms" and a "sick nurse" who received a salary from regular contributions made to the sick fund. These "sick-rooms" were reserved for that use until comparatively recent years. In the Wachovia Historical Museum may be seen an invalid chair which was used for the convalescent patients. It is built of solid walnut, upholstered in leather. No one remembers when the chair was built.

Any attempt at organized nursing should be considered remarkable in those times. Whatever was accomplished was done without conveniences and with only improvised appliances. Had early settlers not been endowed with the true spirit of nursing and the love of the Great Physician, greater numbers of the sick and wounded would have died.

[14] Fries, op. cit., IV, 1717.

CHAPTER II

MILITARY NURSING

THE REVOLUTIONARY WAR

"THE HEROISM of the Revolutionary women has passed from remembrance with the generations who witnessed it: or is seen only in faint and occasional glimpses through the gathering obscurity of tradition."[1] From the scant records scattered here and there a few incidents may be gleaned which throw some light on the conditions of the time. The main impression is one of appalling lack of a sense of responsibility for the care of prisoners on the part of British and American forces alike, and the lack of facilities for even the most primitive methods of housing or nursing the sick and wounded of their own ranks, or supplying the medicines, food, clothing, and small comforts taken for granted in this day.

Dr. Hugh Williamson wrote Dr. Hay on August 24, 1780: "The Articles you was so kind as to order have not been received. Our Hospital patients are near 250, many of them dangerously Wounded. They are lodged in six small wards, without straw or Covering. . . . In the six Wards they have only 4 small Kettles, and no Canteen, Dish, or Cup, or other Utensils. We have hardly any Medicine, not . . . a single Bandage or Poultice Cloath, nor an ounce of meal to be used for Poultices. In a word, nothing is left for us but

[1] Elizabeth F. Ellet, *Women of the American Revolution*, I, 21.

the painful Circumstance of viewing wretches who must soon perish if not soon relieved."[2]

In a further excerpt from *North Carolina State Records* appears this statement: "The Distress this Army has suffered, and still continues to suffer, for want of Provisions. . . . Flour and Rum are the Articles the most in Request in this Climate. . . . Without these, full Hospitals and a thin Army will be all your State or Congress can depend upon in the Southern Department."[3] In Pasquotank County there is among the records an account of Lieutenant Colonel John Patin who, in 1780, had a serious illness and "Constant feavers" which kept him from active duty.[4]

Dr. Williamson wrote to Major England: "I presume that Lord Cornwallis is informed that of the N. Carolina Prisoners lately sent to Charles Town, who I apprehend are from 3 to 400, hardly a single Man has had the small Pox. There is, I presume, the utmost danger of those Men taking the Disease in the Natural way, unless they are inoculated. Be so kind as to inform me whether Lord Cornwallis is willing those Troops should be inoculated and by whom he wishes it should be done." The answer received to the request was very curt, ". . . his Lordship will give proper orders."[5]

Dr. Williamson in correspondence with the Honorable Thomas Benbury from Edenton, on December 1, 1780, related the following: "For eight or ten days after the Battle our people suffered under great neglect. . . . We were also weak in Medical Help. Our Militia Surgeon disappeared after the Battle. . . . It happened one of the Continental Surgeons fell into the hands of the Enemy . . . . tho' he was indefatigable, I found it impossible to give the desired help to 240 Men, who Laboured under at Least 700 Wounds. After three weeks we were happily reinforced by Dr. Johnson a

[2] *North Carolina State Records* (ed. Walter Clark), XV, 61-62.
[3] *Ibid.*, pp. 17-18.
[4] *Ibid.*, p. 22.   [5] *Ibid.*, p. 62.

Senior Surgeon of great skill & Humanity in the Continental Service. . . . We had the misfortune to lose 5 Privates, who died by their Wounds, 9 by Small Pox, 1 by a Putrid fever, and 4 by the Flux; 2 Officers died by their Wounds and 2 by the Small Pox."[6]

The only buildings available for hospitals were churches. At Hillsboro, North Carolina, the *Colonial Records* give an account of an order issued by Dr. Browne, director general of the medical organization, to the quartermaster "to prepare the church as a hospital for the reception of the sick at this point." In another instance the same Dr. Browne wishes to know if he is to "endeavor to fix a Hospital at Hillsboro where I am now going. I have neither money, medicine, nor store with me, and depend altogether on the Consequence yr Letter will give me for supplys. The Legislature of North Carolina will, if you direct me to apply, supply me with medicine there being an apothecary shop at Halifax, which I am told will be seized for my Hospital, provided I procure your approbation." He reported two hundred sick at the post and the number increasing daily. Some of them could have been discharged if clothing and shoes had been available.[7]

In the North Carolina *Gazette,* August 7, 1778, the following advertisement for drugs was found: "Ad. Imported Goods for Sale at Edenton for cash. Senna, jalap, Jesuit's bark, glauber and epsom salts, sarsaperella, etc."

Only an occasional account of nursing done by women of the Revolution can be found, and they appear in heroic light because of the dangers they faced in traveling an unsettled country. North Carolina contributed her share of those courageous souls.

John Motley Morehead III, in *The Morehead Family of North Carolina and Virginia,*[8] describes the great heroism

[6] *Ibid.,* pp. 166-67.   [7] *Ibid.,* IV, 562.
[8] Printed in New York (private printing by the De Vinne Press, 1921).

of Mrs. Kerenhappuck Turner who, when her son went to war, made him promise to let her know if he became ill.

"One of her sons received a fearful wound [he relates]. Word was sent to his mother and she came to him riding on horseback all the way from her home in Maryland. Placing him in a log-cabin on the Guilford Battle Ground, in a crude bed on the floor, she secured tubs in which she bored holes. These tubs she suspended from the rafters and filled with cool water from the 'Bloody Run' which flows nearby. The constant dripping of water on the ghastly wounds allayed the fever and saved her son's life. In this manner did Mrs. Turner improvise a treatment as efficacious as the 'ice-pack' of modern science, and on the spot where this rude cabin stood, the Guilford Battle Ground Company erected a statue in her honor." On the pedestal is the following legend:

A Heroine of '76
Mrs. Kerenhappuck Turner
Mother of Elizabeth
The Wife of Joseph
Morehead of North Carolina and
Grandmother of Captain
James and John Morehead
A young North Carolina soldier under
Greene, rode horseback from
her Maryland home and at
Guilford Court House nursed
to health a badly wounded son

"On Moore's Creek Battle Ground, now National Military Park, stands a monument to the memory of Mary Slocumb, heroine of the battle fought on this ground, and one of the bravest women of the Revolution. This monument was unveiled in August, 1907, with five thousand people present. She was the wife of Lieutenant Captain Ezekiel Slocumb, a Patriotic soldier who lived on the Neuse River in what is now Wayne County. Led by the vision of a dream of a bloody body wrapped in her husband's cloak, she rode all night through the forests of Duplin and Hanover Counties until she heard the roar of battle. Undaunted she went thru the lines. . . ."[9] Seeing a group of men lying under a clump of trees just off the road, she dismounted, fearing to find her husband dead. Uncovering the face of a wounded man, an unrecognized voice begged for water. Picking up a camp kettle, she brought water from a near-by stream. After giving him a drink she bathed his face and discovered he was a neighbor. She dressed a wound on his head and a severe one on his leg, which was bleeding profusely, using a piece of his trouser leg and some heart leaves for a dressing. Then she went from one soldier to another, answering their desperate cries for water and dressing their wounds. While thus occupied, she looked up and there stood her husband, "as bloody as a butcher and as muddy as a ditcher." He had just returned from pursuing the retreating enemy. When the excitement of the glorious victory had somewhat subsided, she again mounted her spirited horse, though in the middle of the night, and made the return trip (in all about one hundred and twenty-five miles) through wild, unsettled, and dangerous country to her home and little child. She is buried near Dudley, south of Goldsboro, beside her husband.

Martha McFarlane Bell was an outstanding figure in the care of the sick near Greensboro. She also acted as a spy for the American forces, under cover of her work as a midwife.[10]

In Robert Henry's account of fighting near King's Mountain, there is an illustration of what seems a unique method of caring for wounds. He says that he continued in extreme pain until his mother made a poultice of wet ashes and applied it to his wounds. This gave him the first relief.[11]

[9] *Greensboro Daily News,* July 5, 1925; see also Ellet, *op. cit.,* I, 361 ff.
[10] *North Carolina Booklet,* XVI, 89.
[11] Lyman C. Draper, *King's Mountain and Its Heroes,* p. 365.

When North Carolina women heard of the deplorable sufferings at Charleston, they "gathered clothing, medicines, and provisions and travelled long journeys." The mother of Andrew Jackson, when on one of those mercy trips, contracted prison fever and died in a tent.

Mrs. David Caldwell of Guilford County has handed down the following relating to the battle of Guilford Court House: "After the wet cold night which succeeded action, the women wandered over the field of battle, to search for their friends, administer the last sad rites of the dead, and bear away the wounded and expiring."

Records show that General Joseph Graham of Lincoln County, North Carolina, was severely wounded by sabre and bullets, receiving four bad wounds on his head and one in his side. He was nearly exhausted from the loss of blood when he reached the home of Mrs. Susanah Alexander where he was "kindly watched and nursed during the night." His wounds were dressed as well as circumstances would permit. He was later removed to a hospital and was two months recovering.[12]

THE CIVIL WAR

"The Civil War marks the beginning of organized concentration of women in this country in public duties."[13] At the outbreak of the war there was no equipment ready for service in caring for the sick. Presumably there had been little inclination to prepare for war in time of peace, even in the midst of rumors of war. Immediately after the declaration of war by the Confederate States of America, military officers were appointed and departments of government organized. The Confederate Medical Department was modeled after that of the Union army. Dr. Charles E. Johnson, surgeon in charge of the State Medical Department, called for volunteers among the women to nurse in the hospitals. Miss

[12] John H. Wheeler, *Historical Sketches of North Carolina*, p. 234.
[13] Mary Adelaide Nutting and Lavinia L. Dock, *A History of Nursing*, I, 357.

M. L. Pettigrew of Raleigh, Mrs. C. C. Kennedy of Wilmington, and Mrs. Beasley of Plymouth were chosen for this great service. A hospital which was prominent during the Civil War was established in Raleigh under the direction of Dr. Edmund Burke Haywood.[14]

Blockade-running was the main source of supply for medicine to supplement the small stock on hand when war was declared. Wilmington was the chief port of departure. As this town was not captured until the fall of Fort Fisher on January 15, 1865, it came to be the only resource of a hard-pressed medical force. The manufacture of drugs from native medicinal plants was encouraged by the State government. Governor Ellis authorized R. B. Saunders of Chapel Hill to open a laboratory for the manufacture of medicine. Blue mass was the chief output. The following advertisement appeared in the Wilmington *Daily Journal*: "Auction Sales—By catalogue—of imported goods." Among the goods are listed ten cases of blue mass at ten dollars a case. Other drugs sold as follows: morphia, fifty-five dollars an ounce; and quinine sulphate, sixty-five to eighty dollars an ounce.[15] A laboratory was established at Lincolnton; and Wilkesboro, Asheville, and Statesville became important collection centers.[16]

The people found substitutes close at hand for many essential articles. Dogwood berries replaced quinine. From blackberry roots and persimmons a cordial was made for dysentery. An extract of wild cherry bark, dogwood, and poplar was a cure for chills and fever. A syrup made from mullein leaves and cherry bark was a remedy for coughs and lung conditions. The castor bean yielded castor oil, and the poppy, opium and laudanum.[17]

[14] Mrs. John Huske (Lucy London) Anderson, *North Carolina Women of the Confederacy*, p. 14.   [15] May 11, 1864.

[16] Joseph Grégoire deRoulhac Hamilton, *History of North Carolina Since 1860*, III, 51.

[17] John Bach McMasters, *A History of the People of the United States During Lincoln's Administration*, p. 335.

On December 2, 1863, the Surgeon General ordered coffee discontinued as an "article of diet for the sick. In consequence of the very limited supply . . . it is essential that it be used solely for its medicinal effects as a stimulant."[18] In 1864 coffee sold for fifteen dollars per pound, and in 1865, for forty dollars per pound.[19]

Homes, churches, and other available buildings were used as temporary bases for hospitals. Such medicines as were brought in by blockade-runners and smuggled through the lines were distributed, when possible, to widely scattered medical units. Quinine in stuffed dolls, emeries, and pincushions made its way to an ague-stricken group of sick here and there. An elaborate funeral was staged in order to get a coffin filled with medicine through the lines. Curtains, carpets, raw cotton, linen, and woolen goods were used for hospital supplies. Public appeal was made for more coverings. Churches, public buildings, and homes were stripped of carpets, which were cut up and made into blankets. Gray moss was used for packing wounds. Horsehair, cotton, or silk thread, when obtainable, served as ligatures. The only methods of sterilization known were charring and toasting. Ambulance service consisted, for the most part, of wagons, carryalls, or improvised stretchers. There was very little comfort for a desperately ill or wounded soldier.

Smallpox existed in many neighborhoods and lesser epidemics were everywhere. In September, 1862, Wilmington was visited by a virulent type of yellow fever. In two months there were 1,505 cases and 441 deaths.[20] There were no trained nurses in the State and very few doctors. A number of Sisters of Mercy from South Carolina, who were sent at the request of the Confederate Government, did gallant and heroic work. New Bern also had a sharp epidemic of yellow

[18] James Ford Rhodes, *History of the Civil War 1861-1865*, p. 367.
[19] Joseph Grégoire deRoulhac Hamilton, *Reconstruction in North Carolina*, p. 77.
[20] Hamilton, *History of North Carolina Since 1860*, p. 51.

fever which occurred during Federal occupation of the town. No statistics are available.

The women who so heroically gave their services in caring for the sick and wounded had no uniforms. It is interesting to note, however, that no bows, hoop skirts, jewelry, or curls were allowed. These workers did not wait to be mustered in, but served under local associations, without pay, as a rule. When appointed by the Confederate Congress, their status was defined as chief matron, assistant matron, and ward matron, and their salaries were fixed at forty, thirty-five, and thirty dollars a month, respectively. The matron was charged with the duties of seeing that the orders of the surgeons were executed, supervising the sanitary and commissary arrangements of the hospital, and satisfying the needs of the individual patients. The actual implication of this last-mentioned duty was described in detail by an experienced matron, Mrs. S. E. D. Smith. "The matron," she wrote, "will call on the steward for whatever diet the patient's appetite calls for, see that it is prepared to suit his taste, feed him herself if he is too feeble to do so; bathe his fevered brow; comb his hair." Other duties enumerated by this same writer included the "dressing of wounds considered too delicate for the hands of male nurses; the placing of pads and pillows so as to relieve the wounds of the patients from the pressure of the mattress; the making of slings and the padding of crutches; the visiting of the wards at every spare moment to join in the conversation of the men, to read and sing to them, write letters for them, and the filling of haversacks when the soldiers returned to the army, or the saying of prayers when death was imminent."[21]

In addition to nursing clubs, hospitals, and aid societies, knitting clubs were organized by churches and communities; these groups worked untiringly far into the night.

[21] Francis Butler Simkins and James Welch Patton, *The Women of the Confederacy,* p. 87.

Churches were used for the storage of the cotton and linen supplies. Women went from house to house distributing this cloth to be made into garments. Sewing machines were scarce in this country and garments such as overcoats, uniforms, and underclothing were often made by hand. They were collected and shipped to some central point of need.

A newspaper of the time, the Wilmington *Daily Journal* of May 28, 1861, printed the following call for volunteer nurses: "To the Ladies. Those ladies who are willing to devote a part of their time to nursing the sick soldiers belonging to the companies stationed at the Marine Hospital, are respectfully requested to hand their names to the undersigned. . . ." Lists of names of women responding from all parts of the State are on record. Particular mention is made of Miss M. A. Buie, "the soldiers' comforter," from Wilmington. Another of the well-known women was Ella K. Newsome, acclaimed by many as "Dixie's Florence Nightingale."

Abby Horne House, affectionately known as "Aunt Abby," has had many tributes paid her. One writer says she was "as fearless under fire as in the use of her tongue" and more than one officer testified to the coolness with which she would walk through the trenches during the fearful bombardment around Petersburg, "frequently going under heavy fire to carry water to our wounded." Though a native of Franklin County, North Carolina, she followed the tide of battle to Virginia and served in the capacity of nurse and general helper wherever she could, with her indefatigable and irrepressible spirit of kindness.[22]

The old Barbee Hotel, now the Arthur, of High Point, was converted into a hospital during the latter part of the war with Laura A. Wesson, a twenty-year-old lass, enrolled as nurse. When a terrible epidemic of smallpox broke out in the hospital, she volunteered to take charge of the "pest

[22] Anderson, *op. cit.*, p. 51.

house." This was an old building, in a field some distance from the town, where the smallpox patients were moved. Laura Wesson nursed them until all were either dead or dismissed. Then she fell a victim of the dread disease and died in April, 1865. Her body now lies in the local cemetery where a monument has been erected to her memory by the Daughters of the Confederacy. Part of the inscription reads, "She fed the hungry, clothed the naked, nursed the sick and wounded, aided by her Father."[23]

Mrs. Elizabeth Carraway Howland, who studied medicine with her father, doctored the Confederate prisoners ill with yellow fever in New Bern. It is claimed that not one of her patients died, though the Yankee doctors lost hundreds. "She was a prison angel secretly clothing and feeding these destitute sufferers."[24]

Mrs. Armand J. DeRosset (Eliza Lord) of Wilmington was a prominent woman of the Confederacy of unusual administrative ability. "While her six sons were fighting, Mrs. DeRosset assisted her husband in his medical work, and nursed the sick, being keenly active to the needy."[25]

Another of the brave, self-sacrificing women of North Carolina who devoted herself to nursing the sick and wounded was Mrs. Jesse (Annie K.) Kyle. Though a frail woman on crutches, she served as head nurse in a hospital at Fayetteville. She had the "indomitable spirit of a lion, working untiringly from early morning 'til night dressing wounds . . . soothing and comforting the dying with Holy prayers," for her prayer book was her constant solace. As other hospitals were established, she answered the calls that were constantly being made upon her, even to following the soldiers to their last resting place.[26]

The home of Mrs. Sarah E. Elliott of Kittrell Springs, a fashionable watering place of ante-bellum days, was con-

[23] Greensboro Daily News, November 14, 1929.
[24] Anderson, op. cit., p. 18.
[25] Ibid., p. 25.   [26] Ibid., p. 40.

verted into a hospital to which were sent hundreds of wounded soldiers. In spite of the excellent care given the soldiers, fifty of them died. Mrs. Elliott and other ladies of this section were untiring in their efforts to relieve suffering, not only with tender nursing, but also with delicacies from their own homes. Mrs. Elliott sent wagonloads of food for their use and encouraged others to do the same.[27]

Tribute should be paid to Mrs. John Harper who gave her beautiful home for the care of the wounded and dying.[28] It was near the site of the battle of Bentonville, which was fought on March 19, 1865.

The sick soldiers in the hospital at Fort Fisher were supplied with nourishing food and nursed by women who courageously remained there. "The wife of Major Stevenson and her sister, Mrs. Mary F. Sanders, were among those who helped to make these Confederates more comfortable, though in constant personal danger themselves."[29] The Soldiers' Aid Society in Wilmington did a wonderful work for the hospitals, supplying clothes, covering, and quantities of provisions.

Mrs. J. Henry Smith of Greensboro tells of the stern reality of the work in that town. Without warning or preparation, wounded soldiers in great numbers were brought there and placed in churches, the courthouse, and every available space in town where beds could be hastily placed. "To that clarion call the women of Greensboro responded with one accord." They nursed the soldiers tenderly and, from their own pantries, fed them. The ill and wounded were later transported to the historic mansion of Edgeworth Seminary which was used as a hospital.[30]

The women of Rowan County did much to relieve suffering among the soldiers. Mrs. Mary A. Wrenn, head of the largest hospital in Salisbury, and her daughter, Miss Betty,

<hr/>

[27] *Ibid.*, p. 45.
[29] *Ibid.*, p. 25.
[28] *Ibid.*, p. 46.
[30] *Ibid.*, p. 57.

worked untiringly. They sold their silver, jewelry, and clothing, as did many others, to buy food for the patients.[31]

North Carolina was quick to adopt from South Carolina the idea of wayside hospitals, which originated among a group of women in Columbia in the winter of 1861-62. These hospitals were hurriedly constructed along the line of railroads at Raleigh, Greensboro, Charlotte, Salisbury, Weldon, Fayetteville, and Goldsboro and were usually maintained by volunteer contributions. They were hastily equipped with medical supplies and crude operating tables.[32]

Among the many who suffered through the scarcity of even ordinary homemade preparations for antiseptic or surgical purposes were the newborn babies and their mothers. Long after the war period, parched flour and scorched bits of cotton or linen cloth were still used for "dressing the baby's cord." These dressings were freshly prepared as needed. The shovel from the fireside was rubbed with ashes and heated before being used as a sterilizing plate.[33]

At the close of the war when the soldiers were being sent home, women continued their services by meeting the passing trains. There they dressed the wounds of the soldiers and provided food for them. Thus with the spirit of the Red Cross, if not the name, these women went through the darkest night and into the most dangerous places to minister to the bodies and souls of the soldiers.

THE SPANISH-AMERICAN WAR

Graduate nurses were given their first opportunity for military service during the Spanish-American War. Although they were inadequately trained or organized for this type of service, the Army and the Red Cross, urged by the Daughters of the American Revolution, decided to give them appointments. The nurses were carefully selected.

[31] *Ibid.,* p. 74.　　　　　　[32] *Ibid.,* p. 15.
[33] *Daily Conservative* (Raleigh), June 3, 1864.

They were required to file a complete record of their professional training and to furnish evidence of good character. When it became known they would receive appointments, the most able leaders in the profession left their post of duty and directed them in war service. During the conflict graduate nurses proved their ability as executives capable of meeting any emergency. Because of more adequate organization the soldiers received better nursing care and the mortality in the army was less than in any of the previous wars.

The following is a list, with all other data that could be secured, of the North Carolina nurses who were appointed for service in the Spanish-American War:

Mrs. Margaret M. Berry, Salisbury, graduate and Gold Medalist of the Maryland General Hospital, Baltimore, Maryland, 1895. Died September 12, 1935, in Washington, D. C. Buried in Hollywood Cemetery, Richmond, Virginia.

Molly Courts, Reidsville, graduate of Retreat Hospital, Richmond, Virginia, 1898. Died February 8, 1935, at Oteen. Buried in Arlington Cemetery, Washington, D. C.

Anne Ferguson, Concord, graduate of Watts Hospital, Durham, 1898. Living in Concord.

Della J. Hall, Salisbury, graduate of Philadelphia General Hospital, Philadelphia, 1895.

Anna D. Schultze, Shelby, graduate of the Philadelphia General Hospital, Philadelphia, 1895.

Lucy Ashby Sharp, graduate of Johns Hopkins Hospital, Baltimore, Maryland, 1895.

Ella Tuttle, Lenoir, graduate of St. Johns' Riverside Hospital, Yonkers, New York, 1896. Served in Jacksonville, Florida, and Cuba. Died April 9, 1934.

Mrs. J. B. McCombs (Dr. McCombs) (nee Farabee Guion), Charlotte.

The World War

Nursing in the World War was done on a gigantic scale. By this time graduate nurse service was well established in the minds of the public. It was taken for granted that the soldiers at home and abroad would be well cared for.

When war was declared the Red Cross took immediate steps to mobilize a vast army of skilled nurses to serve in camps and overseas. Today every Red Cross nurse in North Carolina and elsewhere has a feeling of reverence for Jane A. Delano, director of the National Red Cross Nursing Service. Every nurse who went into the war in any capacity realized that the Red Cross and the United States Government were standing by her and that her needs would be supplied.

At times the nurses endured untold hardships, working endless hours in the barracks and on the firing lines. A small number of North Carolina nurses paid the supreme sacrifice. One died overseas and others were victims of influenza which was sweeping the entire country. Of the nurses who went into service from this state, Dr. Archibald Henderson of Chapel Hill said, "Their names will forever constitute an especial roll of honor." Details of this part of the history are lacking because the nurses are reticent to discuss it, and they were transferred so often and had such varied experiences that it is difficult to get a clear picture of what really took place.

North Carolina, like other states, mobilized units, and got ready to take an active part in the conflict. Dr. John Wesley Long (deceased) of Greensboro organized Base Hospital No. 65 with 32 medical men, 203 enlisted men and 100 nurses; 90 per cent of the nurses were from North Carolina. They were mobilized at one of the nurses' bases in New York City and from there went in a body to France and united with hospital forces at Brest. There they assisted in caring for more than 40,000 patients. Twenty-two hundred desperately ill patients were transported to them before the barracks were ready. There were no electric lights, only oil hand lanterns and flashlights were available. The nurses wore hip boots and waded in slush from building to building. One hundred and two nurses took care of this large number of sick and dying soldiers. Many types of diseases as well as wounds were treated, among which were influenza, pneumonia, pleurisy, cerebro-spinal meningitis, and insanity. In October, 1918, the Chief Surgeon of the American Expeditionary Forces called upon Base Hospital No. 65 for two operating teams to be sent to the front. This was a hazardous duty and called for highly trained women. Dr. Long selected two North Carolina nurses to do this work and they spent many weeks of active service on the firing line and within sound of the "big guns." The work done by this unit has gone down in the history of the War Department as one of unexcelled value. Dr. Addison Brenizer of Charlotte organized an independent unit which later merged with a unit from the Massachusetts General Hospital and formed Base Hospital No. 6.

Excerpts from letters and papers written by a small number of the nurses reveal a few facts about their work. It is found that several North Carolina nurses were members of units in other states. Hettie and Louise Reinhardt of Black Mountain were with Dr. Stuart McGuire's Hospital Unit No. 45. They spent eight months in Camp Sevier, Greenville, South Carolina. From there they were sent to France and worked in Base Hospital No. 87 at Toul. Hettie Reinhardt was acting chief nurse in this hospital until she and her sister returned to the States in 1919. Hattie G. Lowry of Wilmington and Mattie McNeil of Fayetteville were sent out under the American Red Cross Nursing Service with an expedition which had 100 doctors and 1,200 nurses. They were sent to Base Hospital No. 18 but after several changes were attached to Evacuation Hospital No. 3. They worked at Château-Thierry, Toul, and Verdun. They were at Ver-

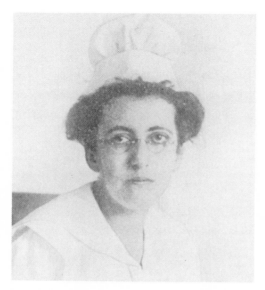

Above, Etta Mae Perkins of Morganton, who died of influenza at Camp Meade. *Below,* Annie Dade Reveley of Greensboro, who died in service in the World War

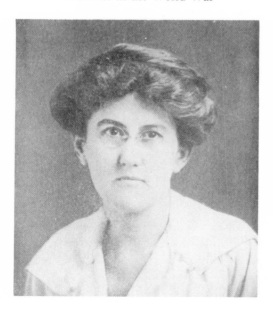

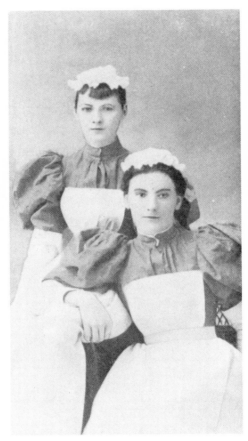

Left, Bessie Mordecai. *Right,* Rosa G. Hill. First graduates of
Rex Hospital

dun when the armistice was signed. These two nurses worked at Treves, Germany, where 1,800 American soldiers were ill and dying with pneumonia and influenza. Elizabeth Clingman (Mrs. W. E. Vaughn-Lloyd), Winston-Salem, served with the University of Maryland Unit.

Mrs. Dorothy Hayden (Mrs. Dorothy Conyers) of Greensboro was a Red Cross Army Reserve nurse in service at Fort Oglethorpe, Georgia, in 1917. From there she went overseas and was in Baccarat, France, in 1918 and Coblentz and other parts of Germany in 1919. Ethel Josey (Mrs. George Hunsucker) of Maiden spent two months at Camp Sevier and, after the armistice was signed, went overseas, December 8, 1918, in a replacement unit. She, with forty others, was sent to Hyères on the Mediterranean Sea to work in a convalescent hospital. Base Hospital No. 99 had arrived prior to this group and had converted six large hotels into hospitals, each a complete unit in itself. Here a large number of patients suffering from tuberculosis, contagious diseases, gas poisoning, and unhealed wounds were cared for.

Ruby Gordon of Biltmore was sent near Château-Thierry and from there to Verdun where the duty of chief of operating rooms was assigned to her. She had five rooms with fifteen tables each running day and night. Often she worked thirty-six to forty hours without rest.

The nurses of North Carolina honor the memory of two of their number who died in service. Annie Dade Reveley of Greensboro, a graduate of St. Leo's Hospital, passed away October 18, 1918, of pneumonia. She was among friends when death came and with military honors was laid to rest in France. Etta Mae Perkins of Morganton, a graduate of Long's Hospital, Statesville, died at Camp Meade, Baltimore, Maryland, of influenza, three weeks after going into service. Cleone Hobbs of Greensboro was with her when the end came. Miss Perkins was buried in Morganton with military honors.

CHAPTER III

HOSPITALS AND SCHOOLS FOR NURSES

THERE WERE comparatively few hospitals in North Carolina before 1900, but after that time they organized rapidly. The early institutions were denominational, state and municipal, and private. The history of only a small number can be given here. The first settlers of North Carolina were for the most part members of the Church of England; therefore, the Episcopalians had a prominent part in building and maintaining the very early hospitals. The Catholics, not so well established, did not sponsor hospitals until 1906. Since then they have built two modern institutions, each with a school of nursing. The first state, municipal, and private hospitals formed the nucleus for several of the largest institutions in the State today.[1]

To encourage young women to prepare for better executive and teaching positions, two North Carolina hospitals offer a course including college work which leads to a B.S. degree and a diploma in nursing. These are Duke University School for Nurses at Durham, and Queens-Chicora College in conjunction with the Presbyterian Hospital at Charlotte. The number of students taking these advanced courses is increasing each year.

A study and comparison of the status of the early hospitals and schools for nurses with those of the present time

[1] See Chapter XI for Negro hospitals and schools for nurses.

will enable the reader to appreciate the rapid progress which has been made.

STATE HOSPITAL FOR INSANE

As early as 1825 the North Carolina General Assembly realized that the care of the insane in North Carolina was very inadequate. Two commissioners were appointed to investigate the plans and expenses of other state institutions and to be prepared to suggest an estimate of the cost of a hospital at the next meeting of the General Assembly.

In 1848 Dorothea Lynde Dix came to North Carolina in the interest of prison reforms. After making a thorough investigation of almshouses and prisons where insane persons and paupers were kept, she found conditions deplorable. In some instances the patients were chained to the floor. The sanitary and housing facilities were as poor in North Carolina as they were in other states. Miss Dix made a detailed report of conditions as she found them and presented it to the General Assembly, asking for an appropriation for a suitable hospital for the care of the insane. Her request met with defeat.

At the time the Assembly was in session, Mrs. James C. Dobbin, wife of the representative from Cumberland County, became fatally ill. Although Miss Dix was not a nurse, she did everything in her power to ease and comfort the dying woman. Mr. Dobbin, wishing to show his appreciation, asked Miss Dix what he could do for her; her request was to help in some way to get funds appropriated for a hospital for the insane of North Carolina. Immediately after the funeral Mr. Dobbin entered the Assembly Hall and made such an eloquent appeal for Dorothea Lynde Dix's request that it was passed overwhelmingly. Thus the General Assembly of 1848 appropriated funds for the hospital and appointed six commissioners to buy not less than one hundred acres of land to be located within three miles of Raleigh. Special taxes were levied to pay for the first buildings, which were to be built of brick.

Miss Dix was given the privilege of suggesting the site for the hospital and the committee proposed that it be named Dix Hill in her honor. This honor she graciously declined, but she asked that it be named in memory of her grandfather, Dr. Elijah Dix, whose one great desire had been to have a medical school in Boston, Massachusetts.[2] A fine portrait of Miss Dix was placed in the reception room as a gift from the State.

Twenty-five years elapsed between the time the hospital was first considered by the Assembly and the time work actually began on the building. Under the capable supervision of Dr. Edmund Strudwick of Hillsboro, the first unit of the hospital was erected to accommodate forty patients. In 1855 Dr. Edward C. Fisher of Richmond, Virginia, was appointed superintendent. The hospital was formally opened February 1, 1856, and twenty-two days later the first patient was admitted. A ventilating system, laundry, workshop, and bakery were installed and improved from time to time. Water was pumped from a reservoir in what is now Pullen Park. From its beginning the institution has been equipped with steam heat.

At the outbreak of the Civil War there were a hundred and seventy-nine patients in Dix Hill. The State not only gave money for the upkeep, but furnished supplies as well. In 1865, when Raleigh surrendered, the federal troops used a large part of the supplies and burned the fences for campfires. When the United States Commanding Officer was notified of this act, he had all supplies replaced and the fence rebuilt.

During the years which followed, many changes were made in the building and equipment. In 1908 the State Hos-

[2] Helen E. Marshall, *Dorothea Dix, Forgotten Samaritan*, p. 119.

pital Commission bought 1,139 acres of land adjoining the original site at a cost of $53,500. This additional land gave opportunity for growth on a large scale. Two colonies were built for epileptics and several buildings were erected for convalescent insane patients. Dr. James McKee was superintendent during this period and was largely responsible for the institution's expansion. Dr. Albert Anderson was elected superintendent in 1913. He instituted vocational training for the patients under the direction of an expert and also installed a complete medical laboratory and dental department.

The school for nurses at the State Hospital was reincorporated as the Dorothea Dix School of Nursing in 1933. Mrs. Myrtle Reams Hall was the first superintendent of nurses, from 1918 to 1926. The student nurses receive two years' training in this large, up-to-date hospital, and in their third year affiliate with a general hospital which makes them eligible for the North Carolina state examinations and for reciprocity with other states. The members of the first class were Kathleen West, Lessie Johnson, and Myrtle Hall. An active alumnae association was organized in 1930.

St. Peter's Hospital

St. Peter's Hospital of Charlotte is the outgrowth of the Charlotte Home and Hospital which was started in two rented rooms on East Seventh Street, January 20, 1876. It was through the vision and efforts of Mrs. John Wilkes, who had her first work in the Charlotte Confederate Hospital, and the members of the Church Aid Society of St. Peter's Episcopal Church that this hospital was established to care for the sick poor of Charlotte. At the end of four months more space was needed. The hospital was moved into a larger house on North Tryon Street. During the first years the hospital was dependent upon individual gifts and donations of every kind for its existence. From the funds raised by the members of the Busy Bee Society, the present site on Poplar and Sixth streets was purchased for $273.42.[3]

The hospital continued to experience financial difficulties for several years and on three occasions was closed for short periods of time. Despite all the discouragements, at the end of ten years two hundred and fifty-four patients had been admitted. In 1885 the city made its first contribution—two hundred dollars.

Work on a new building was begun in 1896, but for lack of funds was not completed until 1898. It was large enough to accommodate twenty pay and ten free patients. The name was changed to St. Peter's Hospital when it was moved into the new building. It was truly a "transformation from a combination poorhouse and hospital" to an "institution where scientific medical care was given patients. . . ." The first X-ray apparatus installed in a North Carolina hospital was placed in this new building.

There were so many calls for trained nurses that a school for nursing was organized in 1899. Ten young women were enrolled in this class and three of them, Susan Mott, Effie Ellen McNeil, and Alice Anna Powers, graduated in January, 1902. A three-year course was given and they were instructed in practical nursing, surgery, materia medica, massage, and cookery.

In 1905 an addition to the hospital was begun, which doubled the capacity, but was not opened for patients until 1907. The hospital was practically rebuilt in 1922 in order to meet the growing demands for more room. The capacity of the present building is sixty-eight patients.

Caroline E. MacNichols, a graduate of West Jersey Homeopathic Hospital, Camden, New Jersey, took charge of St. Peter's Hospital in 1914. She remained there as an able executive until her death in 1932. The nurses who grad-

[3] *Southern Hospital*, Sept. 19, 1936, p. 9.

uated under her leadership placed a memorial tablet in the hospital reception room to show their respect and admiration for her.

Hazel C. Williams has been in charge of the hospital since 1932. The last class of nurses graduated in 1934. There is an active alumnae association.

St. John's Hospital

The members of St. John's Guild, a benevolent organization, were responsible for the establishment of the first hospital in Raleigh in 1878. Through the influence of the Reverend E. R. Rich, rector of the Church of the Good Shepherd, a four-room house was equipped at a cost of $100 and opened for the care of the sick. The treasury contained $67.25 when the hospital was opened. The first matron gave her services in exchange for room and board.

In 1882 St. John's Guild purchased the property on Salisbury Street, formerly the home of Governor Manly, and continued to operate a hospital known as St. John's for a period of ten years. The capacity was sixteen beds. An addition, known as the "Nellie Battle Lewis Memorial Room," built in 1887 by Dr. R. H. Lewis, was designated for the care of sick women who were on charity.

The physicians rendered service faithfully and gratuitously for the sick poor of Wake County. The first attending staff was composed of the following doctors: Peter E. Hines, A. W. Knox, James McKee, R. H. Lewis, and K. P. Battle, Jr. The personnel of the hospital included the Reverend W. M. Clark as chaplain, Maggie McLester as matron, and Jennie Coffin as head nurse.

Rex Hospital

When the will of John Rex, native Pennsylvanian and an early settler of Raleigh, was probated in 1839, it was found that he had left a part of his estate for benevolent purposes. After certain provisions of the will had been executed, there remained a modest sum of money and twenty-one acres of land for the establishment of a hospital "for the sick and afflicted poor of the City of Raleigh."

"The General Assembly of 1840-41 passed an act chartering a corporation to be known as the 'Trustees of Rex Hospital' which was to be managed by five citizens of Raleigh." Those appointed were Judge William H. Battle, William Peace, Thomas J. Lemay, James Litchford, and Richard Smith. The sum of $9,602.06 was left after the stipulations contained in the will had been carried out. The trustees decided to invest the fund in stocks of the State Bank, the Bank of Cape Fear, and bonds of individuals, and by April, 1861, the original fund had increased to $35,262.14. To show their loyalty to the Confederacy, the trustees decided to reinvest the money in Confederate bonds, which soon became practically worthless. After the Civil War they realized what they could from the bonds and in 1893 the fund amounted to about $30,000.00. At this time plans were made to erect a hospital on the plot left by John Rex. This proved to be an unsuitable location and the trustees, by special permission of the court, sold the land for $6,000.00. They purchased St. John's Hospital, August 4, 1893, from the Episcopal Church for $4,500. After building a two-story annex for negroes and making needed repairs, it was opened as Rex Hospital, May 1, 1894, with a matron in charge. The patients were taken care of by ladies in the city who volunteered their services until the arrival of a superintendent of nurses.

In July, 1894, Mary Wyche, recently graduated from the Philadelphia General Hospital, was named head nurse. In October of that year she began the first training school for nurses in North Carolina. Miss Wyche was paid twenty-five dollars per month, with maintenance, for her services as head nurse, bookkeeper, and matron.

When the hospital was opened, members of the Raleigh

Academy of Medicine pledged their services free to charity patients, a service they have continued to the present time.

Rex Hospital was considered an asset to Raleigh regardless of the fact that the furniture and equipment were inadequate. There were no screens for the doors and windows and kerosene lamps and stoves were in use for lighting and heating purposes.

An official report of the hospital in 1904 showed a total of 361 patients admitted, 218 of whom were on charity. The hospital at this time had beds for 40 patients. Several additions had been made to the building during the twenty years it had been in use. The entire plant was valued at $12,647.

In 1896 a childrens' ward was added to the hospital. This was probably the first of its kind in North Carolina. Funds for this addition were solicited by the "Ministering Circle of King's Daughters" with Sadie Tucker as the leader. A much larger ward for children was added in 1923 by W. H. Williamson as a memorial to his wife, Sadie Tucker Williamson. Mr. Williamson also provided an endowment of $10,000 for this ward, and the hospital is now receiving the interest from this money.

The need for a more up-to-date hospital became very evident in 1900 as the present one was housed in a seventy-year-old building and was constantly being repaired. In 1908 the old building was torn away and the cornerstone for a new hospital laid with appropriate Masonic ceremonies conducted by the Honorable Richard H. Battle of Raleigh. It was formally opened to patients in September, 1909. This building, with some changes and additions, served the people of Wake County and vicinity until 1934 when an appropriation for a $397,000 hospital was secured by a Works Progress Administration loan and grant. Mrs. Josephus Daniels of Raleigh, who was a member of the Board of Trustees of Rex Hospital for more than twelve years, went to see President Roosevelt and Mr. Ickes in person and was responsible for the hospital's securing the WPA loan and grant. Later it was found that additional funds were needed to complete and furnish the new building. A campaign to raise $50,000 for equipment was launched by a group of Raleigh men with George W. Geoghegan as chairman. The committee succeeded in raising approximately $25,000. The campaign was then taken over by the Women's Hospital Guild under the leadership of Mrs. Robert Ruark of Raleigh, the president.

Rex Hospital, a new five-story brick building with a capacity of two hundred beds, is ideally located on a nine-acre site on St. Mary's Street. The cornerstone was laid November 15, 1935, and the building opened to patients in May, 1937. The administrator of Rex Hospital is Marcellus Eaton Winston of Youngsville, and the following are the members of the Board of Trustees: Dr. James W. McGee, president; Mrs. Ellen D. Shore, secretary; W. B. Wright; Mrs. C. B. Barbee; and J. W. Bunn, all of Raleigh.

The hospital is modern in every detail. It is the result of the broad vision of John Rex who left a part of his estate to build a hospital for the sick and poor of Raleigh nearly one hundred years ago.

Rex Hospital School for Nurses

The first training school for nurses in North Carolina was organized at Rex Hospital in 1894 under the direction of Mary Wyche, a graduate of the Philadelphia General Hospital, Philadelphia, Pennsylvania. The hospital of only twenty-three beds was rather small to have a school of nursing, but there were patients who needed care, and young women who wanted to be taught the art of nursing.

Five students were enrolled in the first class, but one withdrew to enter a larger hospital in New York. The students living in Raleigh stayed at home and reported at the

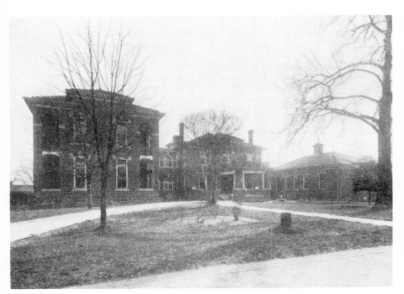

Above, Rex Hospital, Raleigh, 1894. *Below,* Rex Hospital, 1937

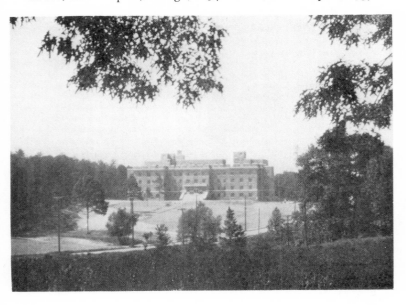

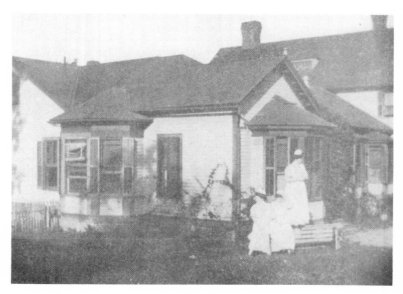

Above, Twin-City Hospital, Winston-Salem, 1895. *Below,* City Memorial Hospital, Winston-Salem, 1938 (courtesy of the Chamber of Commerce of Winston-Salem)

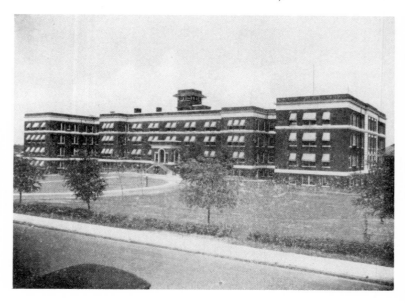

hospital every morning at 8:00 a.m. and remained until 6:00 p.m. They served the first year without remuneration, but the hospital furnished meals and laundry. The first graduating class had two and one-half years of training.

The physicians who assisted Miss Wyche in the training school were Peter E. Hines, A. W. Knox, K. P. Battle, Jr., and James McKee. When the pressure of work was not too great they had classes four times a week in anatomy, materia medica, surgery, obstetrics, and practical nursing. The head nurse was expected to buy any additional text-books she could afford and lend them to the students. The nurses wore regulation uniforms and from the beginning were taught professional ethics. Classes were held in a part of the hospital where the bells could be heard and, if neces-sary, the nurses left the classroom to answer them. It was customary for the head nurse and orderly to care for the patients during class periods.

The members of the first graduating class of Rex Hos-pital were Rosa Gilmore Hill, Elizabeth Mordecai (Mrs. Charles D. Mackey), and Elizabeth Purnell, of Raleigh, and Eva Palmer of Warren County. Miss Hill lives in Raleigh and Mrs. Mackey in Washington, D. C. The other two members of the class are deceased.

From this small beginning, born of necessity, has de-veloped a school which rates as A-1. It has graduated ap-proximately two hundred and four nurses. The school of nursing is under the direction of Lottie C. Corker.

An active alumnae association was organized in 1924 with Mrs. Nora Parks Mimms as the first president. There were thirty-four charter members and it now has an enroll-ment of one hundred and nine.

CITY HOSPITAL OF WILMINGTON

On January 26, 1881, a bill was passed by the North Carolina General Assembly authorizing the County Commissioners of New Hanover County and the Mayor and Board of Aldermen of the City of Wilmington to create a Board of Managers for the City Hospital. This Board was to be organized with suitable officers and regulations governing its actions and was required to furnish both city and county boards with an annual report. After the managers organized and entered upon their duties, they secured a site for the hospital as recorded by a deed in New Hanover County.

Dr. William Walter Lane was elected superintendent and served the hospital until his death in 1901, with the exception of short intervals. The nursing service was done by white and colored women under the direction of Dr. Lane.

The City Hospital continued in operation until the opening of the James Walker Memorial Hospital in 1901.

James Walker Memorial Hospital

James Walker Memorial Hospital was erected upon the site of the old City Hospital of Wilmington in New Hanover County. The building was donated and erected by James Walker, a native of Scotland, for the care of the indigent sick of the city of Wilmington and the county of New Hanover, and such others as might be admitted from time to time under the direction of the Board of Managers. This building was donated by Mr. Walker with the understanding that its management would never enter into politics, that no member of the Board of Managers could be appointed from either the city or county government, and that the city and county would guarantee to appropriate at all times sufficient funds to provide adequately for the care of the indigent sick.

James Walker was a philanthropist and a genuine benefactor. His life's work may be summed up in these words inscribed on the monument erected to his memory in Oakdale Cemetery:

JAMES WALKER

BORN AT DOUGLAS
LANARKSHIRE, SCOTLAND
APRIL 29TH, 1826
DIED MARCH 15TH, 1901
AFTER A FRUGAL AND INDUSTRIOUS
LIFE, HE LEFT TO THE AFFLICTED AND
SUFFERING, A LASTING MEMORIAL OF
HIS BENEFICENCE IN YONDER HOSPITAL
WHICH BEARS HIS HONORED NAME

The hospital, located at Tenth and Rankin streets, was completed to furnish beds for fifty patients and transferred to the city and county Board of Managers of the James Walker Memorial Hospital. The first superintendent of the hospital was Dr. Thomas R. Little. From year to year additions have been made which include a ward of thirty-two beds for colored patients, a five-bed contagious ward, the Marion Sprunt Annex for maternity cases, and children's divisions of thirty-three beds and ten bassinets. A new wing of thirty-eight beds was completed in 1937, making the total capacity of the hospital one hundred and fifty beds.

A charter was granted the James Walker Memorial Hospital on February 5, 1903, to organize and maintain a school for nurses. The first superintendent of nurses was Miss M. Lilly Heller (Mrs. Thomas Little) of Greensboro, and the first graduating class was composed of two members, Florence Hayes (Mrs. Morris Caldwell) of Wilmington, and Alberta Robinson of Dunn. Mrs. Caldwell has the distinction of obtaining the first county certificate of registration issued to a graduate nurse trained in a North Carolina school of nursing. She registered in New Hanover County, July 1, 1903.

An attractive and well-equipped nurses' home was built in 1921 to accommodate 50 nurses. An addition was built in 1937, making 113 rooms for nurses. There are 72 students in the school under the direction of Louise Dimm. Since its organization the hospital has graduated 335 nurses. The alumnae association was formed in 1923 and there are 40 active members.

ASHEVILLE MISSION HOSPITAL

The Mission Hospital of Asheville was established by the Asheville Flower Mission, a branch of the Woman's Christian Temperance Union. In their work of carrying flowers and good cheer to the sick and distressed the women found that the greatest need was not flowers but suitable food and nursing care. It was largely through the efforts of Anna Woodfin, superintendent of the Flower Mission work in Asheville, that the Mission Hospital was organized.

A group of interested women held a meeting in September, 1885, and decided to open a charity hospital. A board of women managers was chosen from the different religious denominations of the town. They rented a five-room cottage on South Main Street and, with the aid of ten dollars a month from the county and provisions sent in by friends, started what is now the largest and oldest hospital in western North Carolina.

The location of the hospital was changed several times during the first years of its existence to meet the demands for more room and better facilities. A report of 1892 gives the total number of patients admitted up to that time as four hundred and seventeen, the majority of them being destitute persons of the city and county. A new building was erected in 1892 and opened for inspection on December 17. A large group of Asheville's oldest and most honored citizens visited and inspected the building. Only a part of it was completed, as funds were insufficient. Interest in hospitals had grown, however, as shown by the memorial beds placed there by different people. The Mission Hospital experienced many financial difficulties and it was still dependent upon gifts from friends and receipts from entertainments. But the perseverance of the Board of Managers and friends resulted in a splendid report ten years after the hospital was opened. From "five rooms and a fund of $10.00" it had grown to a forty-bed hospital. They had cared for approximately one thousand patients.

The first graduate nurse to take charge of the hospital was Elizabeth Spencer of Chicago. The training school for nurses was organized in 1896, and in 1897 the course was increased from eighteen months to two years. The training school was incorporated in 1901 and the period of training increased to three years. A class of three students completed the course in 1899, but did not receive diplomas until 1901.

In 1921 the present fireproof building was started, the old wooden structure having been torn down. The new building opened September 20, 1923. The bed capacity had been increased to 110. The present plant accommodates 125 patients. It is valued at $500,000, and has an endowment of $93,000. A large, attractive, and well-equipped nurses' home was built in 1929 with funds obtained from the estate of Edward Dilworth Latta.

Fannie Vaughn Andrews (Mrs. Duncan Waddill) was superintendent of the hospital from 1917 to 1927. Virginia McKay succeeded Miss Andrews and is still serving in that capacity. There are over two hundred graduates from the school of nursing.

KING'S DAUGHTERS HOSPITAL

In 1887 a group of ten young women of Greensboro organized a club known as "West End." They met twice a month for Bible study and from these meetings developed the idea of contributing to town charities. Although the population of Greensboro was not more than three thousand people, these women realized the urgent need for a hospital. This group joined the National Order of King's Daughters and, with other clubs, set to work to raise the necessary funds for their work. This was done by giving various types of entertainments and by private subscriptions.

Two years later a charter was granted and a lot on Greene Street purchased for $200.00. In 1891 a ten-room house was erected with a Maltese Cross, symbol of the King's Daughters, over the entrance. Mrs. J. O. Hall was the matron in charge of the hospital and the members of the West End Club formed the governing board. The doctors of Greensboro volunteered their services to the charity patients. Due to lack of funds and proper facilities, the hospital closed in 1897. The property was sold in 1917 for $2,000 and the fund given to the Guilford County Tuberculosis Sanatorium.

CITY MEMORIAL HOSPITAL

The City Memorial Hospital of Winston-Salem, with its large buildings, splendid equipment, and spacious grounds, had its beginning in the old Grogan home on North Liberty Street in 1887. A small band of women called a meeting on June 27, 1887, to consider plans for taking care of the needy poor of the community. They met at the home of the late Dr. H. T. Bahnson. Mrs. James A. Gray, Sr., was invited to act as chairman of the committee and to explain the object of the meeting. After a discussion of various types of community work, the idea of organizing a hospital was suggested by Mary Ann Fogle and Maria Vogler, who had done a great deal of work among the poor of Winston-Salem. The idea of a hospital met with the hearty approval of this band of women and they immediately set to work to appoint committees and elect officers who could make plans for financing such a project. The name of this organization was the Ladies' Twin-City Hospital Association.

The first officers elected to serve the association were as follows: Mrs. James A. Gray, Sr., president; Mrs. James G. Buxton, first vice-president; Mrs. J. A. Bitting, second vice-president; Mrs. J. F. Shaffner, treasurer; Mrs. J. M. Rogers, secretary. The first executive board consisted of eleven women selected from the small group who came to this meeting. The president urged this committee to secure a membership of three hundred persons who would pay monthly dues to help get the work started. These members were assessed ten cents a month.

The next meeting was held in the home of the president, Mrs. James A. Gray, Sr., and the treasurer reported that the sum of $83.58 had been collected. This was the fund with which the Twin-City Hospital was started by a group of women who had a strong faith and a real determination to serve those who were unfortunate. The commissioners of Winston and Salem were asked to contribute twelve dollars a month to assist with the care of the charity patients and help pay the rent of a house which could be used temporarily as a hospital.

Six months after the movement for a hospital was started, a suitable location was found, and on December 1, 1887, the Grogan home on North Liberty Street was opened for the reception of patients. The first patient was admitted on December 5, 1887. The efforts of this group of women were looked upon with pride and enthusiasm. By January, 1888, so many gifts were brought in that the pantry shelves were filled. The women furnished milk from their homes.

By 1891 the work had grown so rapidly that the Hospital Association realized the need of a larger building and better equipment to meet the demands of a fast-growing town. After much consideration, a lot was purchased on Brookstown Avenue and a building erected, but it was agreed not to open the new hospital until all debts had been liquidated. The members of the Hospital Association raised funds to erect this building by serving suppers, giving chrysanthemum shows and bazaars, and soliciting donations from private citizens.

The new building was opened October 18, 1895, with Mollie Spach (Mrs. W. F. Miller), a graduate of St. Luke's Hospital, Bethlehem, Pennsylvania, as superintendent. Her services proved invaluable to the new hospital. A training school was not organized for several years, but a small number of young women entered the hospital for one year as helpers and completed their training in northern hospitals.

In 1899 additional rooms and wards were added to the hospital, making a twenty-five bed hospital, and the city was called upon for more financial aid. At this time R. J. Reynolds offered to give the Hospital Association five thousand dollars as an endowment fund if the association could raise a like amount. This was a great undertaking, but it was accomplished by the women of the association, and the benefits of this fund are still being distributed among the needy poor of Winston-Salem. The association decided in 1901 to add a district nurse to the hospital personnel. Her duties were to visit the sick in the community who needed assistance but not hospitalization.

The constitution and by-laws of the hospital were revised in 1901 to provide for a training school for nurses who wished to take a three-year course. Under the leadership of Selena Gilliland, a graduate of the University of Maryland, Baltimore, a class of six nurses was accepted. Three of this number graduated: Laura Crews, Ella Price Smith (deceased), and Ellen S. Watson (deceased).

The work of the hospital increased each year and in 1910 the members of the Hospital Association felt that their work was completed. The pressing need of the times was for a municipal hospital. A site was selected on East Fourth Street and a hundred-bed hospital was erected in 1914. The old Twin-City Hospital on Brookstown Avenue was closed when the City Memorial Hospital was opened.

A nurses' home was erected on the grounds of the City Memorial Hospital from funds received from the former

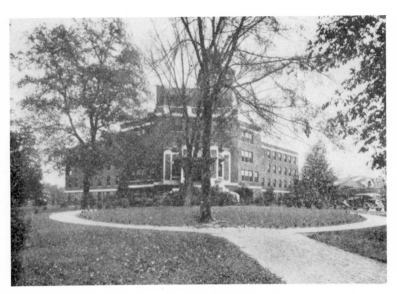

Above, Highsmith Hospital, Fayetteville. *Below,* Watts Hospital, Durham (courtesy of Camera Craft Studio, Durham)

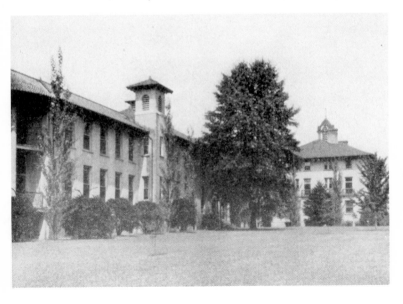

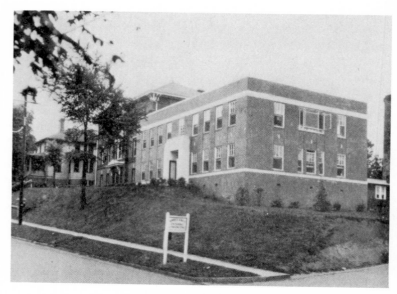

Above, Dr. Henry F. Long's Hospital, Statesville. *Below,* James Walker Memorial Hospital, Wilmington

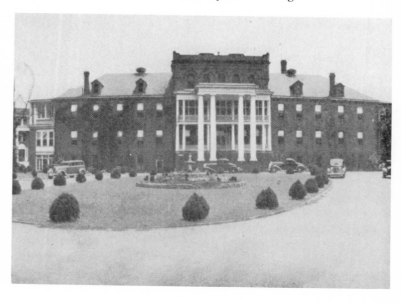

Twin-City Hospital Association. A large brass tablet with a suitable inscription was placed above the mantel in the sitting room as a memorial to the members of the "Ladies Twin-City Hospital Association." In 1930 a much larger and more modern nurses' home was erected from gifts received from Mrs. John Wesley Hanes and Mrs. Robert Edward Lasater, of Winston-Salem, supplemented by funds from the city of Winston-Salem. A tablet was placed in the reception room of the new home in honor of the donors.

Two large additions to the hospital were completed in 1924. One wing was added for colored patients and one for white patients. Two wards for children were included in the new building. A gift of $240,000 from R. J. Reynolds, and $50,000 from Mrs. R. J. Reynolds, of Winston-Salem, and $85,000 from Sterling Smith of Milton made it possible for the city of Winston-Salem to have its present hospital of 225 beds. The hospital also operates a large out-patient clinic.

There are two hundred and thirty-four graduates of the City Memorial Hospital. The alumnae association is very active, having a membership of seventy.

Dr. Henry F. Long's Hospital

Dr. Henry F. Long began the practice of surgery in a private hospital connected with his home in Iredell County in 1891. A graduate nurse, Bettie Walker, was in charge until his sister, Hortense Long, graduated from Atlanta in 1898 and went to work with him. She gave up her duties in the hospital in 1900 to care for their invalid mother. Miss Long died in 1908.

This hospital was the forerunner of the Billingsly Memorial Hospital, which Drs. Long, J. W. Hill, T. E. Anderson, R. M. Adams, and Anne Ferguson incorporated in 1901, with a charter for a training school for nurses. Miss Ferguson was elected superintendent of nurses when the hospital was organized and remained in that capacity nearly thirty-five years. In 1905 Dr. Long moved to his private hospital on Center Street, transferring his school and personnel. The school for nurses was discontinued in 1934 and reopened in 1937.

WATTS HOSPITAL

Through the generosity of George W. Watts, the city and county of Durham received the first unit of Watts Hospital. It was located at Buchanan Boulevard and Watts Street and consisted of an administration building, male and female pavilion large enough to accommodate twenty-two patients, and an operating suite. The hospital and school of nursing were incorporated on February 3, 1895. An endowment fund of twenty thousand dollars was created for the hospital by Mr. Watts. This institution was the first one in the State to benefit from such a fund. The hospital continued its operation in this location fourteen years, during which time the bed capacity had been increased to forty-six.

The present Watts Hospital was presented to the citizens of Durham, December 2, 1909. It comprised four large Spanish-type buildings located on Broad Street in a beautiful oak grove of twenty-seven acres. The capacity of the hospital at that time was ninety beds, but additional buildings erected since 1909 have increased the number to two hundred and twenty-five. Mr. Watts increased the endowment fund from time to time to care for the pressing needs of the institution. The fund now amounts to $500,000 invested in stocks, bonds, and real estate. It is known as the George W. Watts Endowment Fund and the income is perpetual. The hospital is modern in every detail and meets all the requirements of an A-1 institution.

The course of training for student nurses was changed from two to three years in 1908. The first and only graduate of the class of 1897 was Ethel Clay, now Mrs. Julian Price of Greensboro. Mary Wyche served as superintendent of the hospital and superintendent of nurses from 1903 to 1913. Since the organization of the school of nursing, over three hundred graduates have gone out to take their places in the professional world.

The Alumnae Association of Watts Hospital was formed in 1910 and incorporated in May, 1917. There is an active membership of approximately one hundred.

WILSON SANATORIUM

The first hospital established in Wilson was owned by Dr. C. E. Moore and Dr. Albert Anderson and known as the Wilson Sanatorium. The date of its organization was 1896 and the school of nursing was incorporated in 1902. The first superintendent of nurses was Nora Thomas and the members of the graduating class of 1899 were Effie Morris (Mrs. Martin Farotoro), Minnie Oldham, and Annie Morris. Wilson Sanatorium was closed in 1933.

HIGHSMITH HOSPITAL

The Highsmith Hospital of Fayetteville was first incorporated as the Marsh-Highsmith Hospital Company in 1899. It was located on Green Street near the old Market House. The building accommodated fourteen patients. The certificate of incorporation allowed the owners to operate a hospital for the care of surgical and medical patients, to maintain and conduct a school for nurses which granted a diploma for a three-year course, to purchase and sell drugs, and to operate a free dispensary. The hospital and school of nursing have given continuous service since September 1, 1899.

Dr. J. F. Highsmith, Sr., bought the Marsh-Highsmith Hospital Company in 1904 and it was reincorporated at that time as the Highsmith Hospital.

The Cochran Annex was built in 1901 through the generosity of Mrs. Eva S. Cochran of Yonkers, New York. She created an endowment of two thousand dollars annually for the treatment and maintenance of charity patients, both white and Negro. The hospital has received the benefit of this fund over a period of twenty years.

The first class of nurses, graduated in November, 1902, consisted of two members: Mary E. Robinson (Mrs. E. W. Smith of Dunn) and Stella Jones (Mrs. George Weisiger of Fayetteville). Agnes B. Johnson was superintendent of nurses when the first class was graduated.

The present Highsmith Hospital was built on "Haymount," on the corner of Hay Street and Bradford Avenue, in 1926, with a capacity of one hundred and twenty patients. Miss E. A. Kelley, a graduate of Highsmith Hospital, has served as the superintendent of nurses for twenty-five years.

An active and progressive alumnae association organized in 1910 now has a membership of seventy.

MERCY HOSPITAL

In February, 1906, the Sisters of Mercy of the Sacred Heart Convent, Belmont, opened a small hospital with a capacity of twenty beds in an old dwelling house in the city of Charlotte.

There were at that time no members who were trained in the art of nursing, so the Reverend Mother Teresa procured the services of thoroughly trained seculars to aid in the training of Sisters and other students for the work which, at that time, appeared overwhelming. A school of nursing was established. Beulah Squires, a graduate of the University of Maryland Hospital, Baltimore, was the first superintendent of nurses. Sister Mary Bride, Sister Dolores, and Sister Raphael were students in the first class. Ten years later the demand had outgrown the capacity and plans were made for a larger institution.

To Mother Mary Bride, who was then Superior, much credit should be given for undaunted courage and faith, for it was under her leadership that the present hospital was made possible. Ground for this site, at the corner of Fifth Street and Caswell Road, away from the city's noise and dust, yet enjoying all the city's advantages, was given through the generosity of the late Bishop Leo Haid, O.S.B. This, together with the donations and assistance from other influential friends who had observed the work since its inception, made it possible to erect the present hospital, which opened its doors to the public in 1916. The hospital building is entirely fireproof and contains attractive homelike rooms and bright, airy wards for surgical and medical cases, operating rooms, maternity rooms, and a children's department.

Twelve Sisters, nine of whom are registered nurses, give their entire time to this work. A school of nursing education is conducted according to State Board requirements. A new fireproof home for nurses, facing on Vail Avenue, was built in 1922, with a capacity of thirty-five rooms, modern and convenient, with bright class and reception rooms, and a library.

Again in 1930 the demand had outgrown the capacity and plans were made for an additional fifty beds for maternity and infant care. This wing presents the last word in hospital construction and equipment. At present the bed capacity of the hospital, not including bassinets, is one hundred and ten. The hospital is furnished with all the equipment requisite for advanced medical science.

In 1937 an addition to the nurses' home was started and has recently been completed. In this building, also fireproof and modern in every way, are well-equipped classrooms, social and lecture halls, a domestic science room, chemical laboratories, and a library. The grounds are attractive and a splendid tennis court is a popular recreation spot among the students.

On May 26, 1937, the twenty-eighth graduating class received diplomas. The nurses, including Sisters who hold diplomas from Mercy Hospital School of Nursing, number one hundred and thirty-five.

St. Leo's Hospital

Thirty years ago when Greensboro was only a small town, the Sisters of Charity of St. Vincent de Paul of Emmitsburg, Maryland, erected a modern hospital on the corner of Summit Avenue and Bessemer Boulevard. The hospital and nurses' home are built on a ten-acre tract, giving ample space for outdoor activities. The cornerstone was laid on April 26, 1906, two years after the movement for a hospital was started. The original building had a capacity of one hundred beds. An annex was built in 1914 and a splendid nurses' home in 1922, the whole plant representing an investment of nearly a million dollars.

Sister Veronica was the first superintendent of the hospital and Sister Frances Lehey (deceased), the first director of the training school. Sister Regis has given thirty years' continuous service to St. Leo's Hospital. A board composed of the Sisters of Charity governs the policies of this institution.

The school of nursing was incorporated in 1906, and more than two hundred nurses have been graduated from the school. The members of the first graduating class are as follows: Mrs. Dorothy Hayden (Mrs. Dorothy Conyers), Betty Kelly (Mrs. Schenck), Betty Maynard, Miss Hanner, and Miss Manguin. There is an active alumnae association with a large membership.

Duke University School of Nursing

In a codicil to his will in 1925 J. B. Duke requested his trustees to erect and equip a school of medicine, a hospital, and a nurses' home at Duke University. Plans for the organ-

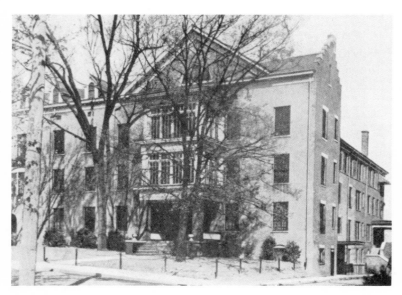

Above, St. Peter's Hospital, Charlotte (courtesy of the Lassiter Press, Charlotte). *Below,* Asheville Mission Hospital

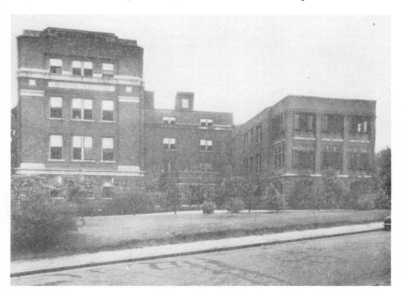

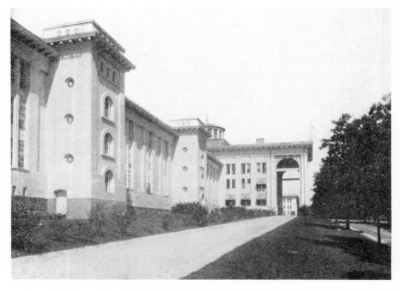

State Hospital for the Insane, Raleigh (courtesy of the
Lassiter Press, Charlotte)

ization of the school of nursing as an integral part of Duke University were started in 1927, and advice in regard to standards in nursing was sought from many sources, particularly from Mary L. Wyche.

On May 19, 1929, the following plan was approved: the granting by Duke University of the Degree of Bachelor of Science to women who have successfully completed two years of college work (60 semester hours) in Duke University or a college or university acceptable to Duke University, and the three-year course leading to the Certificate of Graduate Nurse in the Duke University School of Nursing. The graduates of Duke University School of Nursing, during their three-year course leading to the Certificate of Graduate Nurse, will have completed 70 semester hours of lectures and classes, and 170 semester hours of practical work in wards, diet kitchen, etc. The 60 semester hours of college work can be completed either before or after the course in the School of Nursing. The candidates for the degree of Bachelor of Science are recommended for the degree by the faculty of the School of Nursing and the School of Medicine. Yale and Vanderbilt universities, the universities of Wisconsin and Minnesota, and others have a comparable five-year program leading to the degree of Bachelor of Science. The students in nursing are selected on the same basis as other women students of Duke University; namely, intelligence, character and an acceptable high school certificate.

In April, 1929, Bessie Baker, B.S., R.N., was appointed dean of the School of Nursing and she assumed her duties the following year during the construction of the buildings. The first patients were admitted to Duke Hospital on July 21, 1930, and the first class of the School of Nursing was enrolled in January, 1931. Subsequent classes have been registered each September.

PRESBYTERIAN HOSPITAL AND SCHOOL FOR NURSES

Through the interest of Dr. Elizabeth Blair (deceased), dean of education at Queens-Chicora College, plans were made in 1935 for a combined course leading to a B.S. degree and a diploma in nursing in conjunction with the Presbyterian Hospital at Charlotte. The time required for the course is six years. One nurse enrolled in 1936 and two in 1937. Mary Bell May is superintendent of nurses of the Presbyterian Hospital.

CHAPTER IV

PIONEER NURSES AND LEADERS

IF SPACE permitted, many more North Carolina nurses would find their place among the pioneers. Recent records taken from the clerks of courts throughout the State show that a host of nurses have registered since 1903. Large numbers are still active in some phase of nursing. Among this group are those who have given years of efficient service at the bedside. Many of these have not served as State officers or on committees, but they have been leaders and teachers of good health.

A few years ago nursing was a new profession for women. Training schools had not been established in the South, and those of the North did not appeal to young women of secure social standing. The educated, cultured women from this State who blazed the trail in spite of public opinion and who were not afraid of work or sacrifice deserve credit and honor for their fearlessness. Professional nursing was not established in North Carolina until 1889, but, according to the best authorities, there were three women who went in training from this State prior to that time. They were Jane Christmas Yancey of Warrenton, Fannie Buxton of Asheville, and Evelina MacRae of Wadesboro. Miss Yancey entered Bellevue Hospital in 1877, Miss Buxton the same hospital in 1883, and Miss MacRae the Philadelphia General Hospital in 1884. According to the

reports of this era, graduate nurses were in great demand
and this may explain the failure of these three to return to
North Carolina to practice.

Miss Yancey married Major John Fletcher Harris of Henderson soon after graduation. She died in 1928 at the age of
eighty-one. Miss Buxton nursed in Pennsylvania until her
father's health failed, when she returned to Asheville to be
with him. She died several years ago. Miss MacRae was a
pioneer nurse in Alabama and Pennsylvania. She died in
Philadelphia in 1929.

MARY ROSE BATTERHAM

Mary Rose Batterham was born in England and came to
America when about twenty years of age. After graduating
from the Brooklyn City Hospital in 1893, she went to Asheville, where she did private and public health nursing until
her death in 1928. She had the distinction of being the first
registered nurse in North Carolina and in the United States,
being registered in Buncombe County, North Carolina, on
June 5, 1903.[1] She was a charter member of the North Carolina State Nurses' Association, having attended the meeting
for State organization in Raleigh in 1901. Mary Rose Batterham was a pioneer in her chosen profession, a woman with
a vision for the future of nursing. Her ideals and ethics are
set forth in articles written for nursing organizations. Her
advice to the graduate nurse was to give a day's work occa-
sionally for charity and not to choose her cases. As an educa-
tor she enlisted the interest of nurses in civic needs, welfare
work, the problem of the underfed school child, and the un-
necessary death of mothers and babies. Miss Batterham
advocated shorter hours, improved living quarters, and better working conditions for the student nurse. She felt that
the nurse herself should be a person of superior education
and cultural background; therefore, a broader curriculum

[1] It has recently been discovered that Josephine Burton registered in Craven
County, June 4, 1903.

should be offered during training to produce nurses of the finest type.

ADELINE ORR

Adeline Orr of Brevard was graduated from the Woman's Infirmary, New York City, in 1888. She returned to North Carolina in 1889 and engaged in private duty nursing in Asheville for several years. Upon the completion of the Clarence Barker Hospital, now the Biltmore Hospital, Miss Orr was elected superintendent of nurses, serving in that capacity six years. Her most outstanding work has been done among the women prisoners of Buncombe County in Asheville, where she is affectionately known as "The Angel of Buncombe Prisoners."

Although frail in body, she is strong in character and purpose. With deep compassion for criminals, and the faith of a pioneer, she has wrought many reforms among prisoners. In later years she became interested in the Leprosarium at Carville, Louisiana, and used her time and influence to solicit money for the upkeep of this institution. Miss Orr lives with an invalid sister in Asheville.

MOLLIE E. SPACH

Mollie Spach of Winston-Salem enjoys the distinction of being the first graduate nurse in her native city and among the first to locate in this state. She is a graduate of St. Luke's Hospital, Bethlehem, Pennsylvania, in the class of October, 1889. She returned to North Carolina immediately after graduation and practiced private duty nursing several months. At that time only wealthy patients employed graduate nurses and Miss Spach received many calls from other states, principally Pennsylvania and California. She did not spend a great deal of time in North Carolina until she returned as superintendent of the Twin-City Hospital which was opened on Brookstown Avenue in 1895. She did not have a training school for nurses, but took young women who were interested in learning the profession into the hospital for one year, giving them as much instruction as conditions permitted, and later sent them to northern hospitals to graduate. Miss Spach married W. F. Miller and makes her home in Winston-Salem.

BIRDIE DUNN

Birdie Dunn received her education in the Oxford Seminary, Oxford, North Carolina, graduating in 1895. She chose for her career the nursing profession and entered Bryn Mawr Hospital, Bryn Mawr, Pennsylvania, but later came to Rex Hospital in Raleigh and completed her training in 1898.

Miss Dunn engaged in private duty nursing for twenty years after her graduation. At that time there were very few graduate nurses in the State and she received calls from many people in North Carolina and from other states. After these fruitful years of service she entered a new field of nursing, that of public health, which she has followed for eighteen years.

In 1918 she worked with the Wake County Health Department and in 1919 became affiliated with the North Carolina State Board of Health under the direction of Dr. G. M. Cooper. She is still active in the division of Preventive Medicine and Hygiene.

The Nurses' Relief Fund, established from the sale of Dunnwyche, is a living memorial to the benevolent spirit of Miss Dunn. Her first thought has always been for the sick nurses and especially for those with tuberculosis. She was the founder of Dunnwyche, a home for sick nurses which was established at Black Mountain in 1913 but sold during the World War. Miss Dunn was treasurer of the Relief Fund for a number of years. She has contributed to the growth and development of the nursing profession in North Carolina, being active in state work, serving on the

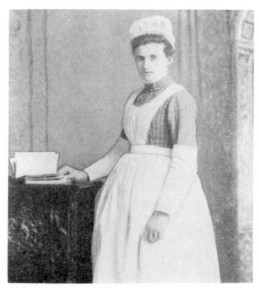

Above, Adeline Orr, graduated from Woman's Infirmary, New York City, 1888. *Below,* Mollie Spach, graduated from St. Luke's Hospital, Bethlehem, Pennsylvania, 1889. These were the first two graduate nurses to practice in North Carolina

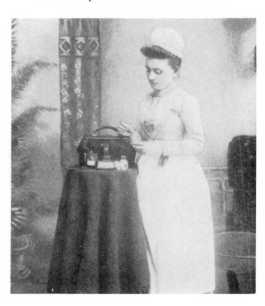

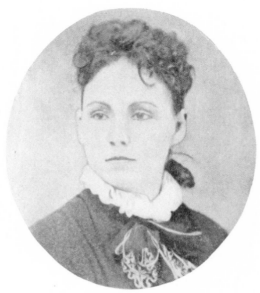

Above, Jane Christmas Yancey, Warrenton, first woman from North Carolina to enter training. Graduated from Bellevue Hospital, 1877. *Below,* Mary Rose Batterham, Asheville. Graduated from Brooklyn City Hospital, 1893. Date of registration, June 5, 1903

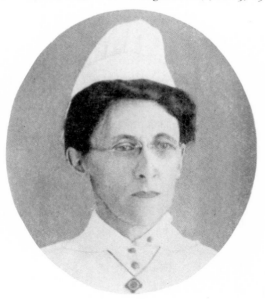

legislative committee over a period of years, and holding offices. She was president of the Raleigh Graduate Nurses' Association twelve years, and secretary-treasurer of Dunnwyche six years. Miss Dunn was one of the fourteen graduate nurses who attended the meeting in Olivia Raney Library in 1902 to organize the North Carolina State Nurses' Association.

Constance E. Pfohl

The first graduate nurse to locate permanently in Winston-Salem and give to the community twenty years of uninterrupted service was Constance E. Pfohl. She graduated from St. Luke's Hospital, Bethlehem, Pennsylvania, on October 18, 1895. She confined her nursing to private duty—much in demand for typhoid fever and other diseases. Several years prior to the influenza epidemic of 1918 Miss Pfohl had retired but she became active again, giving invaluable service during this great scourge. When the North Carolina State Nurses' Association was organized one of the first nurses to be chosen for an important office was Miss Pfohl, a charter member. Her broad vision and clear thinking was of inestimable worth to the association in its formative years. She was elected secretary in 1903 and served faithfully until 1907 and from 1908 to 1913 was president of the State Association. For four years, 1904-1908, Miss Pfohl was president of the North Carolina Board of Nurse Examiners. She organized the first Red Cross Nursing Service in the State in 1910. Since her retirement Miss Pfohl has made her home in historic old Salem where she is closely associated with church and community life.

Nannie Lou Crowson

Nannie Lou Crowson graduated from Rex Hospital in 1897. She engaged in private duty nursing four years. She was a charter member of the North Carolina State Nurses'

Association. In 1901 she married J. R. Jessup and now lives in Fayetteville.

ANNA LEE DE VANE

Anna Lee de Vane was graduated from St. Luke's Hospital, Bethlehem, Pennsylvania, October 18, 1897. After graduation she held the position of superintendent of nurses in the Waterbury Hospital, Waterbury, Connecticut, and Ithaca City Hospital, Ithaca, New York, and was head nurse at the Robert Parker Hospital, Sayre, Pennsylvania. She returned to North Carolina in 1899 and was connected with Dr. J. F. Highsmith's Hospital in Fayetteville for five months as superintendent of nurses. Miss de Vane was better known as a private duty nurse, having spent ten years in active service in Raleigh. In 1917 she returned to St. Luke's Hospital at Bethlehem to take a position as social service worker, and remained there one year. A pioneer nurse in North Carolina, Miss de Vane was active in the work of state organization for graduate nurses. She has the honor of being a charter member of the North Carolina State Nurses' Association. She has served as the first secretary of the North Carolina State Nurses' Association and as a member of the Board of Nurse Examiners. Having retired from active service, she now lives with a sister in Red Springs.

CLEONE E. HOBBS

One of the charter members of the North Carolina State Nurses' Association who has been very active over a period of years is Cleone E. Hobbs of Clinton. She is a graduate of St. Luke's Hospital, Bethlehem, Pennsylvania, in the class of 1897. After engaging in private duty nursing in Bethlehem for a few weeks and executive work in New York for a short while, she returned to North Carolina in April, 1898, to accept the position of assistant superintendent of the Twin-City Hospital of Winston-Salem. She held this position until January, 1900. During this time she relieved the superintendent of the hospital for four months. From Winston-Salem Miss Hobbs went to the State Normal and Industrial College in Greensboro as resident nurse and remained there until May, 1906. In addition to her duties as resident nurse, she was a member of the college faculty the last three years, acting in the capacity of assistant to Dr. Anna M. Gove, who taught physiology and hygiene. The next two years were spent in private duty nursing. Following this, Miss Hobbs accepted a position as superintendent of nurses at the Wilson Sanatorium and remained there two years. From 1910 to 1918 she was engaged in private duty nursing in Raleigh. In 1910 Miss Hobbs became a member of the Red Cross Nursing Service, doing organization work in the State, and later going into active war service for eight months at Camp Meade, Maryland. In 1921 and 1922 she attended summer school at Western Reserve University, Cleveland, Ohio, making a special study of school hygiene. Miss Hobbs was the first nurse selected to serve in the rural counties under the State Board of Health, and she is still active in this work. This appointment was made by Dr. G. M. Cooper of Raleigh. With all the duties of an executive, public health nurse, and private duty nurse, Miss Hobbs found time to serve as a member of the North Carolina Board of Nurse Examiners from 1904 to 1912, being president the last three years, and as president of the North Carolina State Nurses' Association from 1914 to 1916.

Mary Perkins Laxton

Mary Perkins Laxton, daughter of Dr. Joseph Lavender Laxton, prominent physician of Morganton, was graduated from Johns Hopkins Hospital, Baltimore, Maryland, in 1897 and located in Asheville soon after graduation. As a pioneer nurse she was interested primarily in nursing education and in this phase of the profession she has been an able leader in the State.

After coming to Asheville she was engaged in private duty nursing for several years. Her first institutional work was with the Whitehead-Stokes Sanatorium at Salisbury. She assisted in opening this hospital but remained there only a part of one year, after which she returned to Asheville and took charge of Mission Hospital, continuing in this position from 1906 to 1911.

From Asheville she went to the Biltmore Hospital, Biltmore, and for sixteen years was superintendent of nurses and superintendent of the hospital. The first public graduation exercises of these institutions were held under her administration.

For a number of years Miss Laxton was on the Board of Directors of the Associated Charities of Asheville and did active social service work for this organization and for the federal relief which superseded it.

She was president of the North Carolina State Nurses' Association during 1928-1929 and was a member of the Board of Nurse Examiners for eight years, serving as president from 1923 to 1926. From 1930 to 1931 she was executive secretary of the State Nurses' Association, with headquarters in Asheville. In addition to her other activities she has served on many important committees, both state and national. In 1922 she was on the National League of Nursing Education Advisory Council. As a member of the State Legislative Committee she gave generously of her time, and her wise counsel on the problems of the State Nurses' Association has been invaluable.

She now resides with her sister in Asheville.

ANNE FERGUSON

Anne Ferguson of Concord received her training in Watts Hospital, Durham, graduating in 1898. She is a charter member of the North Carolina State Nurses' Association, being one of the original fourteen members who went to

Raleigh in 1901 to assist in organizing the State Nurses' Association. She also has the distinction of being the only graduate of a small North Carolina hospital to receive an appointment from the Army for service in the Spanish-American War. Upon her return from war service in May, 1899, she engaged in private duty nursing in Concord.

In 1901 Miss Ferguson was elected superintendent of Billingsley Memorial Hospital School of Nursing in Statesville. This hospital and Dr. H. F. Long's hospital were merged in March, 1905, to become a private institution. Miss Ferguson continued as superintendent of nurses, serving continuously nearly thirty-five years, retiring in April, 1936, on account of ill health.

As a pioneer in the nursing profession, Miss Ferguson served ably as a leader among hospital executives and over a longer period of time than perhaps any other nurse in the State. Miss Ferguson was secretary-treasurer of the Board of Examiners from 1909 to 1912, a member of the Executive Board of Dunnwyche, and also served as a member of various state committees throughout her years of active service. She now makes her home with her sister in Concord.

Lydia Holman

Lydia Holman, a graduate of the Philadelphia General Hospital, was sent to Ledger in 1900 to nurse a patient with typhoid fever. During the patient's prolonged illness and recovery, Miss Holman made a study of the living conditions of the people and found them lacking in many respects. She became attached to the mountain folk and felt that she could be of help to them in combating disease and in teaching hygiene and dietetics.

After she returned to Philadelphia many letters were received from the people of Mitchell County urging her to come back to them. Miss Holman felt this to be her duty. She availed herself of the opportunities open to nurses for advanced study in slum work and children's diseases and returned to Ledger in July, 1902, as an independent worker. For thirty-seven years she has labored among the people of Mitchell County, helping to reduce maternal deaths, checking the spread of pellagra and many other diseases.

For many years she not only did her housework and cooking, but cared for her horse as well. At any hour of the night she answered the calls of the people, riding alone for miles to attend a person in need. Her arduous duties have been attended by danger and discomforts, by isolation and remoteness from friends, and by the loss of much that makes life enjoyable.

Miss Holman moved from Ledger to Altapass in 1911 and established a temporary infirmary. This property was given by the Carolina Clinchfield and Ohio Railroad.

The Federal Government and the State are taking part in rural public health work at present, with Miss Holman in charge. She was elected a member of the Mitchell County Board of Health in 1936. A public health nurse has been placed in each school in the county to do school inspection work.

L. EUGENIA HENDERSON

L. Eugenia Henderson, formerly of Winston-Salem, now of Charlotte, was graduated from the Maryland University Hospital, Baltimore, in 1901. She returned to her native state and has given to the nurses of North Carolina the value of long years of experience in the nursing profession. She proved her interest in the work of state organization by associating herself with it in the beginning when she became a charter member of the North Carolina State Nurses' Association in 1902.

Salem College, Winston-Salem, chose Miss Henderson as their first infirmarian in 1901 and she remained with them until 1907. Other duties at the college included teaching a class in practical home nursing.

Miss Henderson was among the first graduate nurses at the Twin-City Hospital. She was superintendent of the hospital and the training school for nurses from 1908 to 1913. Her work then was of the pioneer type, as training schools were not well established in the South and required women of ability to make adjustments for a new vocation. Miss Henderson has always stood for the highest ideals in nursing and for better education of the student nurse.

She has spent a number of years in private duty nursing both in Winston-Salem and in Charlotte and is at present actively engaged in this field in the latter city.

Miss Henderson was president of the State Nurses' Association from 1917 to 1919. During this time a training school inspector was appointed and new standards were set up for the schools. She was treasurer of the State Nurses' Association three years, served on the Board of Nurse Examiners from 1912 to 1914, and was a member of several state committees. She has kept abreast of the changes in the nursing world by study and regular attendance at state and national nurses' conventions.

Columbia Munds

Columbia Munds of Wilmington graduated from the Margaret Farmstock School for Nurses in 1902, a postgraduate school connected with the New York Post Graduate Hospital. Her most outstanding service has been with the Wilmington Public Health Nursing Association. It was organized in December, 1918, and she was appointed supervising nurse and is still serving in that capacity.

Prior to 1917 Miss Munds engaged in private duty nursing for several years. In 1917 she developed the Baby Milk Station, at the same time doing hourly nursing. Miss Munds served as president of the State Nurses' Association in 1926 and 1927. She has been a member of several important committees of the State Nurses' Association, among them the Legislative and Relief Fund.

BLANCHE STAFFORD

Truly it may be said of Blanche Stafford of Winston-Salem that she is a "friend to mankind" and a faithful servant to the nurses of North Carolina. Few, if any, have given more years to private duty nursing than she.

For thirty-two years she has engaged in this phase of professional service in Winston-Salem and is still active. The greater part of this time has been spent in doing twenty-hour duty. Miss Stafford entered the University of Pennsylvania in 1902 and was graduated in 1905. She became an active member of the State Association and has served as its president three years, as secretary two years, and has been on the Board of Directors several terms. She was appointed State Chairman of the American Red Cross Nursing Service in 1922 and is still serving in that capacity. While in office as president of the State Nurses' Association, Miss Stafford organized the State into districts. For many years she has been on the legislative committee, giving time, strength, and wise counsel to questions which affected the development of better nursing laws and higher standards for schools of nursing. Miss Stafford worked valiantly to secure rank for nurses immediately after the World War. She helped to raise extra funds for Dunnwyche and served on its Board of Directors.

MRS. DOROTHY CONYERS

Graduating in the first class of St. Leo's Hospital, Greensboro, in 1907 was Mrs. Dorothy Hayden (Mrs. Dorothy Conyers), who soon became a leader in the nursing profession in this State. Her activities in nursing have been diversified. She engaged in private duty nursing nine years, in World War service over two years, and she was Red Cross county health nurse two years. Since 1932 she has been superintendent of the Sternberger Children's Hospital in Greensboro. In addition to her wide experience in the different phases of nursing, she has spent considerable time in study, keeping abreast of the times. This, together with her broad vision and good judgment, has made her an able state officer and committee member.

Mrs. Conyers served the State Nurses' Association as its secretary, 1917-1919; as president, 1920-1921; and as secretary-treasurer of the Board of Nurse Examiners, 1922-1930. She has been secretary of the Standardization Board since 1932. Throughout her professional career, Mrs. Conyers has been interested in furthering the education of both student and graduate nurses, in getting better and more secure legislation, and in raising the standards for schools of nursing.

Essie Alma Kelley

One of the most able leaders among the nurses of North Carolina is Essie Alma Kelley, who came to this state from Union County, Georgia. She was graduated from the Highsmith Hospital, Fayetteville, in 1912, taking postgraduate work in Columbia University and the Pennsylvania Orthopedic Institute. Although the nursing laws were in force and the state organizations in operation when Miss Kelley graduated, she became associated early with state work. The progress of nursing education has been of primary importance to her. The contribution she made in reorganizing the League of Nursing Education and working as its president has been invaluable.

Miss Kelley has been superintendent of nurses of the Highsmith Hospital since 1913. As a state officer she has served in almost every capacity, having been treasurer, 1917-1922; member of the State Board of Nurse Examiners, 1922-1929, and serving as its president in 1929; president of the North Carolina State Nurses' Association, 1929-1931; and president of the Southern Division of the American Nurses' Association, 1931-1933. In addition to holding state offices, Miss Kelley has given wise counsel on many momentous questions relating to legislation, standardization, and relief for sick nurses.

A small number of nurses have gone from North Carolina as missionaries. Their work has been principally as executives and teachers in the hospitals of Africa, Alaska, Korea, and other countries. Information about them is obscure and only a brief review of their work can be given.

Ethel Kestler who graduated in 1903 from St. Peter's Hospital, Charlotte, went to Korea under the direction of the Presbyterian Mission Board.

Mattie S. McNeill, a graduate of the Highsmith Hospital, Fayetteville, went with the Congregational Mission of Durban, Africa, in 1911, in the capacity of charge nurse. She remained in the Mission Hospital at Durban for three years.

Lossie de Rosset Cotchett (Mrs. Richard Lynch), a member of the James Walker Alumnae Association, was sent by the Episcopal Church as a missionary nurse to St. Johns in the Wilderness, a mission station inside the Arctic Circle. She and a deaconess were the only white people in the station. At the end of the first year Miss Cotchett was transferred to a mission school at Nenana. After working in the mission field five years, she married Richard Lynch and they live at Anchorage, Alaska.

Nina Lewis Farmer, who was graduated from the Presbyterian Hospital in Charlotte in May, 1919, received her appointment from the Southern Mission Board in June, 1920. She sailed October 9, 1920, for Mutoto Station, Africa. She spent nearly ten years in the Congo Mission at the Goldsby-King Hospital. An excerpt from a letter written by an intimate friend says of Miss Farmer, "Her duties reached from the missionary families to deserted native orphans; from the Bible school where she taught classes, and played the organ for songs—the hospital where she helped the doctors in every way; to the inmates of the filthy jungle huts, where

on her bicycle she often answered the cry of suffering natives
. . . ." She died March 12, 1931, following an operation and
is buried at Mutoto Station, Africa.

Two members of the City Memorial Hospital Alumnae
are in the foreign field. Blanche Hauser of Forsyth County
went to Korea in 1923. She is now a member of the staff of
the Union Medical College, an institution for doctors and
nurses located at Seoul. Prior to this year she was superintendent at the Methodist Hospital at Wonsan.

In 1936 Laura Mosley went to Nicaragua under the auspices of the Home Moravian Church of Winston-Salem.

Mamie Thomas of Winston-Salem went to Guinhagak,
Alaska, August, 1928, as a missionary under the auspices of
the Home Moravian Church. She returned to North Carolina in 1933.

Mrs. Mary L. Yorke, one of the early graduates of the
Twin-City Hospital, Winston-Salem, is superintendent of
the Alaskan Moravian Orphanage at Bethel, Alaska. She has
held this position since 1930.

CHAPTER V

NURSING ORGANIZATIONS

The North Carolina State Nurses' Association

THE NURSES of North Carolina are indebted to Mary Lewis Wyche, who was the leader in the organization of the State Nurses' Association.[1] It required much patience and persistence to overcome the timidity of the nurses and to stimulate enough interest to get them together to make plans for a state organization. The small group of pioneer nurses who came to the first meeting in Raleigh in 1901 cannot be honored too highly. They were women who had the vision and foresight to build a solid foundation even though there was much opposition to their plans.

Miss Wyche attended the meeting of the International Council of Nurses in Buffalo in 1901 and heard discussions on legislation and registration. She was impressed by the discussions and was conscious of the need of legislation for nurses in North Carolina. Upon her return to the State she made plans to get the nurses together to form a State Nurses' Association. At that time superintendents of nurses scarcely knew each other by sight and were too busy to get acquainted. In private duty the isolation was even greater, as the nurses were usually on duty twenty-four hours a day. She felt that their greatest need at that time was for an organization that would bring them together in a social way,

---

[1] For list of charter members, see Appendix A, p. 135.

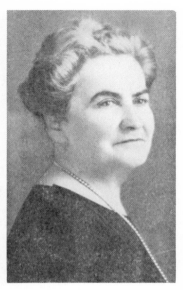 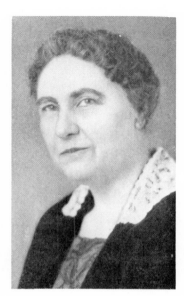

Upper left, Mary Lewis Wyche, first president of North Carolina State Nurses' Association, 1902-7. *Upper right,* Constance E. Pfohl, second president, 1908-13. *Lower left,* Cleone E. Hobbs, third president, 1914-16. *Lower right,* L. Eugenia Henderson, fourth president, 1917-19

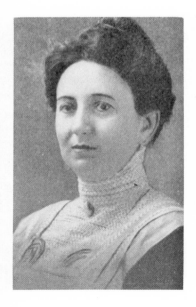 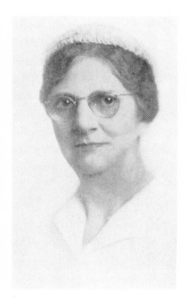

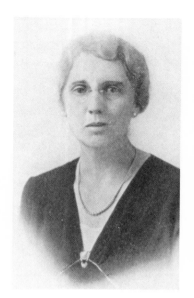 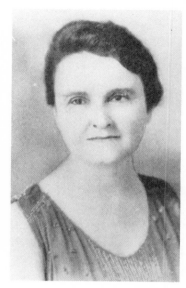

Upper left, Blanche Stafford, fifth president of North Carolina State Nurses' Association, 1920, 1924-25. *Upper right,* Dorothy Conyers, sixth president, 1921-22. *Lower left,* Pearl Weaver, seventh president, 1923. *Lower right,* Columbia Munds, eighth president, 1926-27

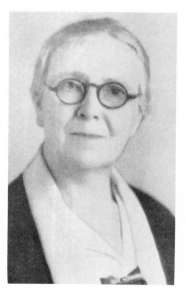 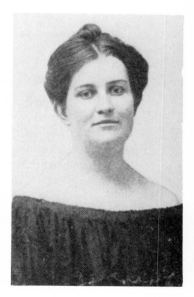

and through which the nurses of the State could formulate and work out plans for the upbuilding of the profession. In October of that same year she gave expression to this belief when she sent out postal cards to the Raleigh nurses with the following request:

"Please meet me at the office of Dr. A. W. Knox at four o'clock P.M. Wednesday, October———1901. MARY L. WYCHE." Not a nurse responded, but she was undaunted by this lack of interest and two weeks later sent out a second postal card to the nurses with a notice which read:

"There will be an important meeting of the Raleigh Nurses' Association at 4 o'clock P.M. Wednesday, at Dr. A. W. Knox's office.

October———1901   MARY L. WYCHE."

Her perseverance was rewarded this time and every nurse was present, eager to know what the Raleigh Nurses' Association was, and what had been done at the previous meeting. She confessed the ruse she had used to bring them together, and then unfolded her plans for an organization of nurses in Raleigh and asked their opinion. A Raleigh Nurse Association had been formed previously but for lack of interest had disbanded. They were enthusiastic over the idea of forming a new association and immediately set out to make the second attempt a reality. The interest grew with each succeeding meeting and before spring it was found that this enthusiastic little group of nurses was planning the organization of a state association.

They sent questionnaires to every nurse in the State whose address could be secured, asking the following questions: "Do you approve of state organization for nurses? Do you approve of state legislation for nurses? Do you approve of state registration for nurses?" The mails brought slow but favorable replies, and with this encouragement they made plans to invite the nurses from all over the State to meet with them in Raleigh, Fair Week, October 28-29, 1902. This week was chosen because of the special rates the railroads were offering, and the attractions other than a get-together of the nurses.

In response to the invitation, fourteen nurses arrived for the meeting which was held in the assembly room of the Olivia Raney Library, October 28, 1902. Mary Rose Batter-ham of Asheville was made chairman, and Annie Sturgeon of Raleigh, secretary pro tem. Miss Wyche was asked to state the object of the meeting. A condensed report of this meeting is as follows:

There were three definite objects, as stated in the questionnaires, which Miss Wyche explained in detail and discussion began at once. An outline of the work, together with the proposed constitution and by-laws, presented and adopted on the second day, follows:

"Article I. This Association shall be known as the North Carolina State Nurses' Association.

"Article II. The objects of this Association shall be the organization and registration of nurses, the advancement of all interests which appertain to the betterment of the nursing profession. And to establish a professional reciprocity between the nurses of North Carolina and nurses of other states and countries. Also to secure legal enactment regulating professional nursing.

"Article III. Officers. The officers of this Association shall be a president, first vice-president, second vice-president, secretary and treasurer.

"Sec. 2nd. The control and management of this Association shall be vested in a board of directors.

"Article IV. Amendments. This constitution may be amended by a two-thirds vote of the members present at any regular meeting, provided such proposal has been submitted in writing at a previous meeting, or thirty days notice thereof shall have been mailed to each member, by the secretary.

Miss S. A. HAYES
Miss NANNIE LOU CROWSON
Miss ANNE FERGUSON"

The election of officers was by nominations from the floor. The following nurses were the first officers of the State Association: Mary Lewis Wyche of Raleigh, president; Mary Rose Batterham of Asheville, first vice-president; Annie Sturgeon of Raleigh, second vice-president; Anna Lee de Vane of Red Springs, secretary; and Miss Z. B. Henderson of Raleigh, treasurer.

Miss Batterham made the motion that the president appoint the chairman of the standing committees and that the chairman be allowed to select her assistants. This motion was carried, with the results as follows: Anna Lee de Vane of Red Springs, printing; Ella Case of Asheville, membership; Mrs. Marion H. Laurance of Raleigh, ways and means. A motion was made and carried that all moneys be deposited in the Raleigh Savings Bank. By a unanimous vote it was decided to hold the first annual meeting in Asheville, June 9, 1903.

The Association was incorporated under the laws of North Carolina, December 5, 1902, and the following is a copy of the Certificate of Incorporation:

"THIS IS TO CERTIFY, That we, Mary L. Wyche, Mary D. Pittman and Marion H. Laurance and associates do hereby associate ourselves into a corporation, under and by virtue of the provisions of an act of the Legislature of the State of North Carolina, Session 1901, entitled 'An act to revise the Corporation Law of North Carolina,' and the several supplements thereto and acts amendatory thereof.

"FIRST: The name of the corporation is North Carolina State Nurses' Association Company.

"SECOND: The location of the principal office in this State is at No.———Street, in the City of Raleigh, County of Wake.

"THIRD: The objects for which this corporation is formed are to organize and register nurses; the advancement of all interests which appertain to the betterment of the nursing profession, and to establish a professional reciprocity between the nurses of North Carolina and the nurses of other States and countries; also to secure if possible legal enactment regulating professional nursing. Only white nurses shall become members of this Association. The corporation shall also have power to conduct its business in all its branches, have one or more offices, and unlimitedly to hold, purchase, mortgage and convey real and personal property in any State, Territory or Colony of the United States and in any foreign country or place.

"FOURTH: The names and post office address of the incorporators are as follows:

NAME	POST OFFICE ADDRESS
Mary L. Wyche	Raleigh, N. C.
Mary D. Pittman	Raleigh, N. C.
Marion H. Laurance	Raleigh, N. C.

"FIFTH: The period of existence of this corporation is limited to 60 years.

"IN WITNESS WHEREOF, We have hereunto set our hands and seals the Fifth day of December, A. D. nineteen hundred and two.

MARY L. WYCHE
MARY D. PITTMAN
MARION H. LAURANCE

Witness
W. M. RUSS

STATE OF NORTH CAROLINA   } ss.
COUNTY OF WAKE

"BE IT REMEMBERED, That on this the Fifth day of December, A. D. nineteen hundred and two before me, a Clerk of the Superior Court, personally appeared Mary L. Wyche, Mary D. Pittman and Marion H. Laurance, who I am satisfied are the persons named in and who executed the foregoing certificate, and I having first made known to them the contents thereof, they did each acknowledge that they signed, sealed and delivered the same as their voluntary act and deed, for the uses and purposes therein expressed.

W. M. Russ
Clerk of Superior Court

(Official Seal)

Filed Dec. 5th, 1902
J. BRYAN GRIMES,
Secretary of State

STATE OF NORTH CAROLINA
OFFICE OF SECRETARY OF STATE

"I, J. Bryan Grimes, Secretary of State of the State of North Carolina, do hereby certify the foregoing and attached (two (2) sheets) to be a true copy of the Certificate of Incorporation of North Carolina State Nurses' Association Company and the—probates thereon, as the same is taken from and compared with the original filed in this office on the 5th day of December A.D. 1902.

"In Witness Whereof, I have hereunto set my hand and affixed my official seal.

"Done in office at Raleigh, this 5th day of December, in the year of our Lord 1902.

J. BRYAN GRIMES,

(Seal)   *Secretary of State"*

From this modest beginning, the nurses have seen their profession advance to a place of importance in the State and in the nation.

The State Nurses' Association, which became a member of the American Nurses' Association in 1918, is now composed of five sections; namely, the league of nursing education, private duty, public health, office, and industrial nursing, each meeting the requirements of the American Nurses' Association. At the annual meeting of the North Carolina State Nurses' Association each section contributes to the well-planned and instructive program.

THE BOARD OF NURSE EXAMINERS

The Legislature of 1903 passed a law creating a Board of Nurse Examiners to be composed of two physicians, elected by the North Carolina Medical Society, and three registered nurses from the North Carolina State Nurses' Association. The first physicians who served on the Board were John Wesley Long of Greensboro and R. S. Primrose of New Bern. The first nurses who represented the North Carolina State Nurses' Association on the Board were Constance E. Pfohl of Winston-Salem, Mrs. Marion H. Laurance of Raleigh, and Mary L. Wyche of Durham. The election of these members took place at their respective state meetings in June. On December 16, 1903, the Board met in Greensboro for the purpose of perfecting its organization. At this time Miss Wyche explained the object of the meeting, and after a free discussion by the various members of the group in regard to the standards they desired to inaugurate, they arrived at the conclusion that the advancement of nursing education and the encouragement of state registration should be their first objective.

The following is a copy of the by-laws adopted by the Board of Examiners at a call meeting in Greensboro, November 22, 1904:

"Article I, Sec. I—Election of Officers: The following officers shall be elected by ballot, a majority vote deciding the election: a president, secretary and a treasurer—these officers to serve during this membership on the Board.

"Article II, Section I—Duties of Officers: The president shall preside at all meetings of the Board and shall perform all duties incident to that office.

"Section II—The secretary shall keep a correct record of all the meetings of the Board. She shall give to the public press notice of the meetings of the Board, and shall attend to all correspondence of the Board.

"Section III—The treasurer shall have charge of all moneys of the Board, shall keep a correct account of all sums received and disbursed, and shall pay no bills except upon written order signed by the president.

"Committees

"Article III, Sec. 1. The president shall appoint such committees as, in the wisdom of the Board, seem necessary.

"Voting

"Article IV, Section I. Voting for the election of officers, the application for license as Registered Nurse and the revoking of license as Registered Nurse, shall be done by ballot.

"Amendments

"Article V, Sec. 1—The by-laws may be amended or new by-laws enacted by a majority vote of the board.

"Amendment of June 23, 1909

"No nurse is eligible for examination who has more than four months of unfinished time in her three years' course even though the hospital sees fit to issue a diploma."

The following officers were elected: Mrs. Marion H. Laurance, superintendent of Rex Hospital, Raleigh, president; Mary L. Wyche, superintendent of nurses, Watts

Hospital, Durham, secretary-treasurer. Mrs. Laurance died in September, 1904. Constance E. Pfohl of Winston-Salem was elected president at a call meeting held November 22, 1904, to fill Mrs. Laurance's unexpired term.

The first examination was held in Raleigh, May 24, 1904. Certificates were issued to Hattie Lowry and Ida Thompson, Watts Hospital, Durham; Edith M. Redwine, St. Peter's Hospital, Charlotte; Julia Stinson (Mrs. W. S. Pharr), Myrtle Hawkins, and Celeste Bell (Mrs. S. A. Stevens), Presbyterian Hospital, Charlotte.

Each member of the Board selected his or her subject for examination. The time and place of meeting was the same as that of the Medical Society since the railroads gave them special rates. The members of the Board paid their expenses to the first meeting as there were no funds in the treasury until 1905.

The work of the Board of Examiners of Trained Nurses has proved to be a most important step in the educational advancement of nurses in the State. Its influence upon the curriculum has done much to give the schools a recognized educational standard.

The laws were revised in February, 1917, and the name changed from the Board of Nurse Examiners to the Board of Examiners of Trained Nurses in North Carolina. The name was again changed in 1931 to North Carolina Board of Nurse Examiners.

At a joint meeting in Greensboro, December 3, 1923, of special committees appointed by the North Carolina Hospital Association and the North Carolina State Nurses' Association, it was unanimously agreed that one physician on the Board of Examiners of Trained Nurses in North Carolina be appointed from the State Medical Society and one from the North Carolina Hospital Association.

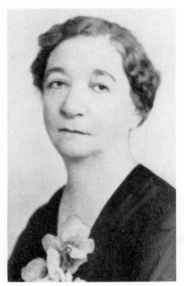
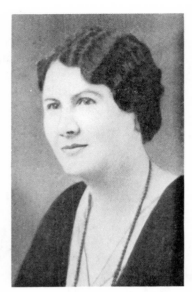

Upper left, Mary P. Laxton, ninth president of North Carolina State Nurses' Association, 1928-29. *Upper right,* Miss E. A. Kelley, tenth president, 1930-31. *Lower left,* Hettie Reinhardt, eleventh president, 1932-34. *Lower right,* Ruth Council, twelfth president, 1935-37

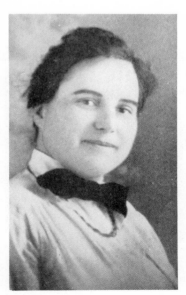
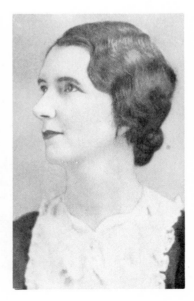

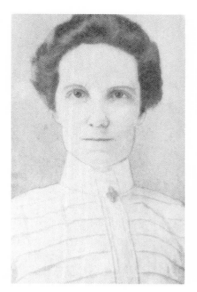 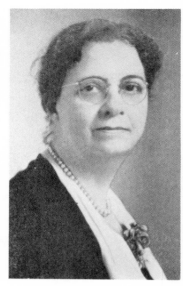

Upper left, Mrs. Marion H. Laurance, first president of North Carolina Board of Nurse Examiners. *Upper right*, Mrs. E. Irby Long, present president of North Carolina State Nurses' Association. *Below*, first Public Health Nurses, 1918. *Reading left to right*, Birdie Dunn, Cleone Hobbs, Mrs. H. P. Guffy, Flora Ray, Cora Beam, Katherine Livingstone

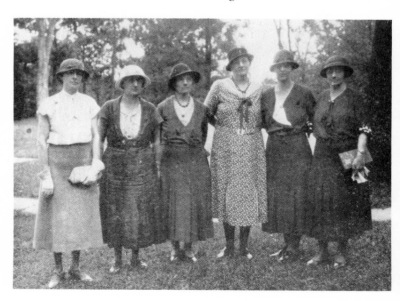

The League of Nursing Education

At a meeting of the North Carolina State Nurses' Association at Asheville in 1910, an organization known as "The Association of Superintendents of Hospitals and Training Schools" was formed with seven members. The following officers were elected: Mary Laxton, president; Mary L. Wyche, first vice-president; Ella H. MacNichols, second vice-president; Mary Helen Trist, secretary and treasurer.

The association planned to meet annually with the State Nurses' Association and to pay dues of one dollar a year. A constitution and by-laws were not adopted at the time of organization. There were not enough nurses of this group present at the 1911 state association meeting to make any future plans. According to the Minutes of 1912, "The Association of Superintendents of Hospitals and Training Schools" asked to have the name changed to "Educational Section" and to include in its membership head nurses and surgical nurses. After this was done a round-table discussion followed which dealt primarily with the better education of the student nurse. Particular interest was shown in a uniform curriculum and standard textbooks for each school, the length of the probation period, and the vacation of the student nurses. Each year the study of the problems vital to the training schools was continued and at the State meetings programs and discussions were held relative to their solution.

When the North Carolina State Nurses' Association convened in Winston-Salem in 1916, the members of the Educational Section discussed the advisability of organizing the North Carolina League of Nursing Education in accordance with the laws of the National League of Nursing Education. A committee was appointed with Katherine Rothwell (deceased) as chairman and Miss E. A. Kelly as secretary. This committee kept busy and at the State meeting in Kinston in 1918 their plans materialized and the North

Carolina League of Nursing Education, with Edith M. Redwine as president and Miss E. A. Kelley as secretary, was
organized as a section of the North Carolina State Nurses'
Association. There were twelve charter members. They
outlined a four months' preliminary course for probationers,
and suggested having classes during the day instead of night
classes, as had been the custom. Even though the superintendents of the hospitals realized that their methods were
inefficient and proposed the changes, it was not easy to
adjust the work to meet the new requirements.

In 1920 the North Carolina League had twenty-five
members. At an enthusiastic meeting in Charlotte the fol-
lowing papers were read and discussed: "How May the
Eight-Hour Day be Established in the Average Hospital?";
"Modifying the Standard Curriculum to Meet the Needs of
the Average Hospital"; and "Arranging Class and Lecture
Work to Fit in with the Routine of Ward and Nurses
Hours."

Effie Cain, secretary of the Board of Nurse Examiners,
advocated definite educational requirements for entrance
into nursing schools. She said the schools were not demand-
ing proof of one-year high school education, which was the
interpretation of the law at that time, and some nurses
had been refused State examinations on this account. Miss
Burgess, president of the National League of Nursing Education, in her address in 1929, said, "The States were not en-
forcing the good legislature they had secured in the early
years."

The members of the League of Nursing Education continued to suggest changes which they felt would be beneficial to the schools of nursing. During 1923 Miss E. A. Kelley
of Fayetteville instituted practical examinations which were
given in addition to the regular examinations by the State
Board of Examiners. They also recognized the fact that the

overworked superintendents of nurses needed whole-time instructors for the students. Many of them arranged to send some members of their graduate staff to Columbia University to take postgraduate work. These nurses returned with a real sense of responsibility for the better education of the student nurse. By close coöperation with the North Carolina Hospital Association recently organized, the League of Nursing Education was greatly benefited. Through this organization the hospital administration and the members of the League obtained mutual understanding of many of their problems.

The practice of student nurses' going from one school to another was becoming more or less general. The League made a recommendation to the Board of Examiners that a student nurse spend at least two years in the school from which she received her diploma. At present very few superintendents will receive a student from another school unless it has been discontinued and the student is recommended by the State Educational Director.

Presidents who served the North Carolina League of Nursing Education so ably during its early years were Mary Laxton, Gilbert Muse, and Virginia McKay. Under their leadership instructive programs were arranged and presented at the State nurses' meetings. Among the subjects discussed were "Recreation for Student Nurses," "Modified Student Government," "Arrangements of Daytime Classes," "Teaching of Practical Nursing," and "Instructors in Schools."

Under the capable leadership of Miss E. A. Kelly from 1927 to 1929, a complete reorganization of the League was effected. Changes were made in the constitution and by-laws to conform to those of the National League of Nursing Education. Another forward step was the financial support it gave to the Grading Committee.

Although the North Carolina League has always been composed of a small group of nurses, it has manifested great interest in the educational growth of hospitals and nurses generally. In 1925 it sponsored a three-day institute which was held in Asheville and conducted by Mary C. Wheeler of Chicago. The charges were nominal and many nurses availed themselves of this splendid opportunity to become more familiar with the solutions of their problems. Another institute, lasting three days, was held in Durham in 1928 and was conducted by Margaret Carrington of Western Reserve University.

At a meeting of the North Carolina Hospital Association in 1929 the League of Nursing Education presented a plan showing the advantages of graduate nurse service over the student plan in the small hospitals where the education of the nurse is difficult and expensive.

Meetings have been held jointly with the North Carolina State Nurses' Association each year and educational programs have been arranged for each session. Growth in numbers has been very slow, but interest in the work has always been evident. In 1933 the constitution and by-laws were again revised to meet the requirements of the National League of Nursing Education. Announcement was made that psychiatric clinics were being conducted at Dix Hill in Raleigh for the benefit of student nurses.

The North Carolina League has made every effort to keep abreast of the advancement made in nursing education. One-day institutes have been conducted by many of the districts and considerable time has been given to the study of the latest changes in the *Curriculum Guide* for student nurses. In 1936 and 1937 an institute lasting two weeks was conducted at Chapel Hill with Lelia I. Given, instructor of Nursing Arts, South Dakota State Teachers College, as teacher.

Bessie Baker, dean of the School of Nursing, Duke University, has been president of the North Carolina League of Nursing Education since 1935.

RED CROSS NURSING SERVICE

In the spring of 1910 Jane A. Delano, president of the American Nurses' Association and director of the National Red Cross Nursing Service, requested Constance E. Pfohl, president of the North Carolina Nurses' Association, to organize a state Red Cross nursing committee at the next annual convention of the State Nurses' Association. This meeting was held in Asheville in June, 1910, and the subject was discussed but, as little enthusiasm or interest was displayed, nothing definite was done at that time.

At a meeting called by Miss Pfohl at Greensboro in the fall of 1910, plans were made to organize the first state Red Cross nursing committee. Miss Pfohl was elected chairman and secretary and the following nurses served with her: Mary Wyche, Raleigh; Ella MacNichols, Charlotte; Cleone Hobbs, Greensboro; and Hattie Lowry, Wilmington. Appointments for membership on state and local committees have always been made by the National Red Cross Nursing Service at Washington, D. C. The first local Red Cross nursing committee for the purpose of enrolling nurses was organized in Winston-Salem in 1911.

The first enrolled Red Cross nurses in North Carolina formed the first State committee and were appointed as follows: Constance E. Pfohl of Winston-Salem, chairman and secretary, April 27, 1912, to September 22, 1914, reappointed July 2, 1918, and resigned September, 1922; Mary Wyche, Durham, May 28, 1912, served until 1922; Ella MacNichols, Charlotte, February 2, 1911, served until December, 1919; Cleone Hobbs, Greensboro, May 28, 1912, became chairman and secretary, 1916, and resigned in September, 1918, to go into World War service; Hattie G. Lowry, Wilmington, July 19, 1916, served until 1918; Florence M. Perry, Wilmington, April 27, 1912, served until her death in 1916; Mrs. Dorothy Hayden (Mrs. Dorothy Conyers) of Greensboro, September 19, 1914, served until 1918, reappointed, and served in 1921 and 1922.

The Winston-Salem local committee enrolled the nurses in the western part of the state, and Wilmington enrolled those in the eastern section. North Carolina had eighteen enrolled nurses in 1913 but the membership had increased to twenty-eight in 1914.

The two active Red Cross nursing committees in the State in 1914 were in Wilmington and Winston-Salem. The Wilmington committee was composed of the following: Hattie G. Lowry, chairman; Margaret J. Graham, secretary; Sibbie Kelly, Gertrude Petteway (deceased), Stella Pettway, and Mrs. Grace Hengeveld. The Winston-Salem committee was composed of the following: Constance E. Pfohl, chairman; Percy Powers, secretary; Sallie Hardister, Hallie Kuykendall, Mamie Thomas, and Elizabeth Clingman (Mrs. W. E. Vaughan Lloyd).

Miss Hobbs made every effort to recruit an emergency detachment of ten Red Cross nurses for the Mexican Border trouble in 1915. She was unable to secure that number as there were only seven nurses in the State who could meet the requirements of the American Red Cross.

Four Red Cross nurses were appointed to serve during the Confederate Veterans' reunion at Jacksonville, Florida, in 1915. They were Cleone Hobbs of Greensboro, Mamie Thomas and Sallie Hardister of Winston-Salem, and Mary Wyche of Henderson.

Hettie Reinhardt of Black Mountain volunteered for service in a unit organized in 1915 by the National Red Cross Headquarters and sailed for Russia on March 20, 1915. She was appointed for service in an eight-hundred-bed hospital, under the auspices of the Russian Red Cross, remaining there six months. When Mrs. Helen Scott Hay, chief nurse of this unit, was transferred to Serbia, Miss Reinhardt was assigned to relieve her. This work was discontinued October, 1915, because of the strained relations existing incident to the World War. After her return to America, Miss Reinhardt was informed that she would be decorated for her services by the Imperial Russian Government but, due to the immediate fall of the government, the decoration was not given.

The entrance of the United States into the World War caused the National Red Cross Nursing Service to waive the former requirements for Red Cross enrollment. North Carolina had not been able, on account of its small hospitals, to graduate nurses who qualified for Red Cross enrollment; thus the number did not increase from twenty-eight until after 1916.

Miss Hobbs, who was active in the private duty nursing field, kept up the work of State organization and enrollment. In June, 1917, she organized a local committee at Charlotte. Julia Lebby and Ella MacNichols were appointed as members. Greensboro and Raleigh were organized in March, 1918, and Asheville, in August, 1918.

The number of Red Cross nurses increased rapidly and the State was able to send one hundred and eleven into military service, either in camps or overseas. Miss Hobbs resigned to enter the World War service at Camp Meade, Baltimore, Maryland. Constance E. Pfohl was again reappointed as chairman and secretary on July 2, 1918. In 1921 North Carolina had a membership of two hundred and sixty-two Red Cross nurses.

Classes in home hygiene and care of the sick were taught in 1917 at Gastonia, Greensboro, Raleigh, Tarboro, Shelby, and Wilmington.

The National Red Cross Nursing Service was advised of

Lelia M. Idol's appointment as a member of the Winston-Salem local Red Cross nursing committee through a letter from the Southern division office, dated July 8, 1920. On September 23, 1920, the Southern division in Atlanta informed the National Red Cross Service of her appointment as secretary of this committee, and she continued in this office until December 28, 1929, when she resigned as secretary but still continued to serve on the Winston-Salem local Red Cross nursing committee. Through all these years Miss Idol was greatly interested and very loyal and rendered most efficient service. On June 24, 1927, Miss Idol was appointed a member of the North Carolina State Red Cross Nursing Committee and served until 1933.

Following the war there was a period of reorganization of Red Cross activities in the State. A number of the nurses had enrolled but had not returned to North Carolina; others were still abroad doing rehabilitation work; thus the necessity of revising the committees and the enrollment in 1920.

Blanche Stafford of Winston-Salem, who was appointed State chairman on September 19, 1922, is still serving in a capable and efficient manner.

The Greensboro local committee was discontinued in July, 1923, and the Asheville committee, November 1, 1924. This territory was assigned to the Winston-Salem committee. On April 25, 1927, the Raleigh committee was discontinued and Winston-Salem and Wilmington took over their work. The Asheville committee was reorganized on April 28, 1927, with Jane Brown as chairman.

In 1938 North Carolina has four local committees for enrollment of Red Cross nurses, located at Asheville, Charlotte, Raleigh, and Winston-Salem. The total membership is three hundred and fifty-four.

Eleven Red Cross nurses in North Carolina were called for service during the Ohio and Mississippi Valley flood of 1937. Five were assigned from Charlotte; namely, Ida Reid Cohen,

Lillian Faires, Naomi Moore, Louise Mason (Negro), and Lillian Jenkins (Negro); and six from Winston-Salem, Ruth Council, Nell Davis, Mildred Foreman, Mary Lofton, Beatrice Long Solomon, and Ethel Shore.

The North Carolina State Red Cross Nursing Committee in 1938 is as follows: Blanche Stafford, Winston-Salem, chairman and secretary; Lillian Bagley, Jane M. Brown, Asheville; Lottie C. Corker, Raleigh; Marie A. Farley, Goldsboro; E. A. Kelley, Fayetteville; Columbia Munds, Wilmington; Lucy Price, Charlotte; Mrs. Willie B. F. Raulston, Greensboro; Lucy Royster, Durham; S. Evelyn Smothers, Winston-Salem; Hazel C. Williams, Charlotte.

PROFESSIONAL REGISTRIES

The organization and maintenance of professional registries in North Carolina has not been phenomenal, but they mark the trend of progress of nursing activities in the State.

In 1932 the Board of Directors of the American Nurses' Association applied the term "official" to all registries meeting the following requirements: "The official registry in a given community is that registry which has been so designated by the local District Nurses' Association, and has been approved as such by the State Nurses' Association. Where there is no District Nurses' Association, the State Nurses' Association is to approve and designate the official registry."

In 1937 the term "official" was replaced by "professional" according to the ruling of the Board of Directors of the American Nurses' Association.

The list of professional registries, registrars, and date of organization found in North Carolina is as follows:

NAME OF REGISTRY	REGISTRAR	DATE ESTABLISHED
Asheville Directory for Trained Nurses	Mrs. Daisy D. Ambler, R.N.	1921
Charlotte Nurses' Official Registry	Nida Cook	1921

Greensboro Nurses' Directory	Mrs. Madge L. Abercrombie	1926
Raleigh Nurses' Registry	Della Wheelers, R.N.	1935
Wilmington Official Registry, District No. 9	Lillian George, R.N.	1912
Winston-Salem Official Registry for Nurses, District No. 2	Mrs. Mary R. Gladstone, R.N.	1930

THE PUBLIC HEALTH SECTION

A small group of public health nurses responded to the invitation of Dr. L. B. McBrayer to meet at the State Sanatorium, April 6-7, 1916, to consider organizing a Public Health Section. This group of twelve nurses formed an organization with Percy Powers of Winston-Salem as chairman. They applied for membership in the State Nurses' Association as a Public Health Section. After some discussion they were accepted as an affiliated branch for one year, later becoming a regular section of the State Association. In 1917 they conducted a round-table discussion of their problems at the State convention. At this time they elected Mary Rose Batterham chairman. During the following years much was done to stimulate interest in this section through well-planned programs on tuberculosis, nutrition, school child welfare, family case work, immunization, midwives, and venereal disease control.

Among the leaders of this group who have served as chairman of the section are: Rose M. Ehrenfeld of Raleigh, Katherine Myers of Charlotte, Clara Ross of Tarboro, Columbia Munds of Wilmington, Mrs. Blanche T. Lambe of Greensboro, Lucia Freeman (deceased) of Fayetteville, Ruth Council of High Point, Marie Farley of Goldsboro, and others. The number of public health nurses has grown steadily. In 1924 there were forty-five; in 1930, ninety-four; and in 1937, approximately two hundred.

The Private Duty Section

The Private Duty Section of the State Nurses' Association became active in 1917 according to the minutes of the State convention. Hattie Lowry of Wilmington was chairman. The large number of nurses who comprise this section have been primarily interested in the distribution of nurses, in group and hourly nursing, and in the organization of professional registries. During periods of economic stress they have adjusted hours and fees to help meet the situation.

In recent years representatives from the American Nurses' Association have been invited to speak to the private duty nurses on eight-hour duty. Very little has been accomplished. Members of Districts Nos. 7-9 at Fayetteville and Wilmington, respectively, have been doing eight-hour private duty nursing in the hospitals for the past two years.

Among the nurses who have served as chairman of the Private Duty Section are the following: Mattie Moore and Estelle Torrence, Charlotte; Mary C. Oldham, Greensboro; Blanche Stafford and Lucille Cain, Winston-Salem; Olivia Ericson, Asheville; and Katherine Goodman, Raleigh.

Organization of the Districts

Prior to August, 1919, the graduate nurses of North Carolina had been organized into groups known as local nurses' clubs. These clubs were located in the larger towns throughout the state. Later when the American Nurses' Association required the State to be divided into districts, these clubs formed the nucleus of the district headquarters. Blanche Stafford of Winston-Salem, president of the North Carolina State Nurses' Association, made a tour of the State, visited the different local clubs, and explained the new plan which was to go into effect in the other states. The former locations of the nurses' clubs throughout the State were selected as centers for the districts, and the counties most accessible to them were incorporated to form that particular district.

The following is a list of the districts, with date of organization and the counties comprising it:

Asheville Nurses' Association, 1919, District No. 1—Avery, Buncombe, Burke, Cherokee, Clay, Graham, Haywood, Henderson, Jackson, Macon, Madison, McDowell, Polk, Rutherford, Swain, Transylvania, and Yancey.

Winston-Salem Nurses' Association, 1920, District No. 2—Alleghany, Ashe, Davidson, Davis, Forsyth, Rowan, Stokes, Surry, Watauga, Wilkes, and Yadkin.

Charlotte Nurses' Association, 1920, District No. 3—Alexander, Anson, Cabarrus, Caldwell, Catawba, Cleveland, Gaston, Iredell, Lincoln, Mecklenburg, Stanly, and Union.

Greensboro Nurses' Association, 1920, District No. 4—Alamance, Caswell, Guilford, Montgomery, Randolph, and Rockingham.

Durham Nurses' Association, 1920, District No. 5—Chatham, Durham, Granville, Orange, and Person.

Raleigh Nurses' Association, 1920, District No. 6—Franklin, Johnson, Vance, Wake, and Warren.

Fayetteville Nurses' Association, 1920, District No. 7—Bladen, Cumberland, Harnett, Hoke, Lee, Moore, Richmond, Robeson, Sampson, and Scotland.

Wilson Nurses' Association, 1920, District No. 8—Beaufort, Bertie, Camden, Chowan, Currituck, Dare, Edgecomb, Hyde, Lenoir, Martin, Nash, Northampton, Pasquotank, Perquimans, Gates, Green, Halifax, Hertford, Pitt, Tyrrell, Washington, Wayne, and Wilson.

Wilmington Nurses' Association, 1920, District No. 9—Brunswick, Carteret, Columbus, Craven, Duplin, Jones, New Hanover, Onslow, Pamlico, and Pender.

THE STANDARDIZATION BOARD

The Standardization Board was created for the purpose of working with the Board of Examiners of Trained Nurses in North Carolina in outlining standard requirements by which the schools of nursing could be graded on their individual merits. The members of the Standardization Board, appointed in May, 1925, were as follows: Drs. J. B. Whittington of Winston-Salem, chairman; B. C. Willis of Rocky Mount; C. M. Strong of Charlotte; J. M. Parrott of Kinston, honorary member; and Mrs. Daisy D. Chalmers of Asheville; Catherine McDuffie of Fayetteville; Lula West of Mt. Airy; and Hettie Reinhardt of Winston-Salem, secretary.

Lack of funds prevented the North Carolina State Nurses' Association from having an educational director for three years. In 1925 they asked Lula West of Mt. Airy to make a six weeks' survey of the schools of nursing in order that a report could be made of the conditions under which student nurses were being trained.

The Standardization Board used this report and recommendations made by former educational directors as a basis for a schedule of minimum requirements for the classification of schools of nursing. In outlining the requirements the members of the Board considered that educational advantages of the student, textbooks used, hours on duty, and living conditions were of vital importance. Dr. Whittington urged them to set a high goal and he is in a large measure responsible for the present requirements for accredited schools of nursing in North Carolina. A copy of the requirements was sent to every hospital in the State.

A questionnaire was sent to each school of nursing and from these the Standardization Board hoped to gain knowledge of the efficiency of each hospital which was privileged to send out young women as graduate nurses. About two thirds of the hospitals participated in this movement. According to the standards set up by the committee, each school of nursing would automatically grade itself as A, B, C, or D classification. The schools falling in any one of the four classes were recognized for two years. After that time D was eliminated, and at the end of three years, C and D were not allowed to take the North Carolina State Board examination.

Dr. Whittington resigned as chairman of the Board in 1927. Hettie Reinhardt was elected secretary for a term of three years. Other changes in the personnel of the Board were as follows: Dr. J. T. Burrus (deceased) of High Point became chairman; and Dr. B. F. Royal of Morehead City, Columbia Munds of Wilmington, and Elizabeth Hill of Statesville became members.

The schools of nursing were graded by the questionnaires received and a report sent to each hospital. An added requirement was that a graduate of dietetics teach the subject. A committee was appointed to ascertain if affiliation with hospitals within the State could be established.

In 1931 the members of the Standardization Board were very much concerned about the oversupply of nurses and suggested to the schools of nursing that they use a ratio of one nurse to three patients, abolish the use of student nurses for special duty, and close small schools of nursing. As a result of the 1930 survey, the schools were reclassified.

Virginia McKay of Asheville and Dr. Duval Jones of New Bern were appointed to serve on the Board in 1931. In 1932 Mrs. Dorothy Conyers of Greensboro was elected secretary and Dr. J. F. Highsmith of Fayetteville, chairman. Other members added were Dr. W. N. Thomas of Oxford and Dr. G. L. Carrington of Burlington. In May, 1937, the following were elected to serve as members of the Board: Dr. Hiram Lee Large of Rocky Mount; Dr. Harry Lester Johnson of Hickory; Newton Fisher, superintendent of James Walker Memorial Hospital, Wilmington; and Dr. Carrington, who was reëlected to serve three years.

THE OFFICE NURSE SECTION

In 1930 Miss E. A. Kelley of Fayetteville was appointed chairman of a committee to make a survey relative to the number of nurses engaged in office nursing, and their interest in organizing an Office Nurse Section. Her report was given at the State Nurses' Convention in 1930 and a section was organized with Mrs. Walter Denmark of Goldsboro as chairman. Due to the limited number of nurses participating in this branch of nursing it ceased to function after the first year. It was reorganized at the State Nurses' Convention held in Wilson in 1936 with Nola Currie of Charlotte as chairman.

THE INDUSTRIAL NURSE SECTION

The Industrial Section of the North Carolina State Nurses' Association was organized in Winston-Salem, May 20, 1937. The following officers were elected: Mrs. Louise P. East of Albemarle, chairman; Lillian Tilley of Greensboro, vice-chairman; and Louise Shelton of Winston-Salem, secretary. This section was the last in the State to organize but the number of industrial nurses is increasing rapidly and they represent an important phase of the profession from an economic as well as humanitarian standpoint.

Among the corporations which are employing graduate nurses are R. J. Reynolds Tobacco Company of Winston-Salem; Chatham Manufacturing Company of Elkin; Wiscassett Mills, Incorporated, of Albemarle; Enka Corporation of Enka.

CHAPTER VI

STATE EDUCATIONAL DIRECTORS

AT A CALL meeting of the Board of Examiners held in Asheville, October 12, 1915, Lois A. Toomer, a graduate of the James Walker Memorial Hospital at Wilmington, was appointed training-school visitor. Her duties consisted of visiting the training schools of North Carolina and obtaining an accurate knowledge of their standards and working conditions. For this service she was allowed three dollars a day and traveling expenses. She was instructed to show each school wherein it was lacking in organization and courses of study, and to discuss the decision of the Board of Examiners with the schools relative to future eligibility of nurses.

The first report submitted by Miss Toomer showed that there were thirty-nine training schools in the State. Fourteen of this number had fifty or more beds and three had less than fifteen. She also found that pupil nurses were being sent into the surrounding vicinities to take care of serious cases of illness without supervision or regard to the length of time spent away from classes. Other defects in the organization of the training schools were their failure to keep records of the students' work and the lack of uniformity in the textbooks used.

After the Board of Examiners heard Miss Toomer's first report it decided to outline a systematic course of instruction and to require uniform textbooks to be used by the schools.

During the Legislature of 1917 the nursing laws were revised and a provision made for a training school inspector to be appointed annually by the State Nurses' Association. A survey of the schools was not made in 1917 due to pending legislation.

From 1917 to 1922 Edith M. Redwine of Monroe, a graduate of St. Peter's Hospital, Charlotte, was inspector of schools of nursing and during her term of office made a complete survey of the schools. In the *Transactions* of the Sixth Annual Meeting of the North Carolina Hospital Association of May, 1923, may be found an article entitled "A Plea for Training School Standardization," in which Miss Redwine gives a detailed report of the survey. Her recommendations for better standards are as follows:

"1. A general classification of hospitals and training schools as A, B, C, and D, according to equipment, class and number of patients treated, character of work done, and manner of meeting requirements.

"2. More and better qualified teachers in our schools of nursing.

"3. Better lighted, ventilated and equipped class and demonstration rooms.

"4. Uniform curriculum and standard text-books arranged to meet state needs and requirements.

"5. Whole-time instructors or teaching supervisors to teach, supervise study hours and give more attention to the practical work of the students.

"6. More correlation in theory and practice.

"7. Longer service in dietetics, obstetrics, and pediatrics.

"8. A better method of teaching dietetics in the majority of schools. [The problem might be solved by the co-operative dietitian, employed jointly by two or more hospitals in a community to teach theory and some practice, giving an equal number of days to each hospital and co-operating with the housekeeper for the application of theory to practice.]

"9. Some practical work as well as theory in mental nursing, tuberculosis and orthopedics.

"10. Less time devoted in schools of nursing to special branches, such as X-ray, anaesthesia and laboratory work unless the student wishes to specialize, in which case it should be elective the last six months.

"11. A standardized unit system to comprise one year high school.

"12. More graduate nurses (at least two) on the staff of every accredited school of nursing.

"13. Regular and uniform class time, possibly nine months, though the present classification is not significant." [More and better work is often accomplished in a six or seven months' term systematically planned than in a longer period with lectures and classes constantly omitted on the slightest pretext.]

"14. Systematized class work and study hours.

"15. Uniform minimum and maximum allowance.

"16. Transfer system from one school to another for those students wishing to make a change.

"17. Less routine hour work, except what is necessary to instruct the students and give satisfactory service to the patients under their care.

"18. More thorough teaching in probation period of personal and household hygiene and practical nursing procedure.

"19. Thorough teaching of ethics and nursing history, state laws and requirements.

"20. Good reference libraries containing latest books on nursing subjects, nursing and hospital magazines and instructions in how to use.

"21. Non-employment at least on same footing, as licensed nurse, of those who have not complied with state laws relative to registration.

"22. Affiliation arranged to meet services required.

"23. A more nearly equalized service in departments for the individual student. [Use of students in this way may partially explain the tendency among nurses to specialize, of which we hear so much complaint. The nurse only knows how to do the thing which she has had to do.]

"24. A simple but complete record of the students' time, work and deportment.

"25. Provision of wholesome amusements at the hospital."

These recommendations and others form the basis of those later set up by the Standardization Board and today are recognized as the minimum standards for an accredited school of nursing.

Due to insufficient funds the office of educational director was discontinued from 1922 to 1928.

Lula West, graduate of St. Vincent's Hospital, Norfolk, Virginia, former superintendent of nurses of the Martin Memorial Hospital of Mt. Airy, was elected in 1928 as state educational director. She served as secretary-treasurer of the North Carolina Board of Nurse Examiners beginning in 1932. While she was in office an annual survey was made of all the schools of nursing in the State and a detailed report given at each State meeting. During the time that Miss West was educational director many improvements were made in the schools of nursing throughout the State. Old hospitals were enlarged and new ones built. There was increased interest in nursing education. Entrance requirements had been raised, better class rooms provided, more whole-time instructors employed, the number of graduate supervisors increased, carefully planned curriculum used, and the students' records were in much better condition. There were a number of new homes built for nurses, the old ones were enlarged and improved, and facilities for recreation added. Many small hospitals closed their schools of nursing and employed a graduate nursing staff.

In 1936 Bessie Chapman, graduate of Memorial Hospital in Richmond, Virginia, was elected to fill the position of State educational director made vacant by the resignation of Miss West, as well as the unexpired term of secretary-treasurer of the North Carolina Board of Nurse Examiners. A permanent office has been established in Raleigh with headquarters for the State educational director. Miss Chapman was elected secretary-treasurer of the North Carolina Board of Nurse Examiners in 1937 for a term of three years.

CHAPTER VII

LEGISLATION AND REGISTRATION
FOR NURSES

NORTH CAROLINA has the distinction of being the first state to secure registration for nurses. This bill was passed and signed by Governor Charles B. Aycock on March 3, 1903. The purpose of the bill was to secure for future nurses better education in theory and such skill in practice that the public would have confidence in the registered nurse. North Carolina was the first state to make an amendment to the nursing laws.

Mrs. Marion H. Laurance, superintendent of Rex Hospital, was appointed chairman of the first legislative committee, but a few days later asked to be released. Miss Wyche took her place. Honor is due the members of the legislative committee of the North Carolina State Nurses' Association who had the foresight and courage to prepare a bill for registration. With the State Nurses' Association less than one year old, these wide-awake women, with the aid of friends among lawyers and doctors, framed the first bill entitled, "An Act to Provide for State Registration for Trained Nurses in North Carolina." The bill was presented to the General Assembly of 1903 by John C. Drewry, "the gentleman from Wake." It is as follows:

"Section 1.—That after Jan. 1st, 1904, any nurse who is not less than twenty-three years of age, and holds a certificate of training in an incorporated general hospital, showing that he or she has had not less than twelve lectures from the Medical Staff or Superintendent during each year of his or her training; or in a hospital or sanitarium, provided the hospital is a general one and not special, that is, one which accepts and treats medical, surgical and obstetrical cases; or holds a certificate of two years training, in theory and practice, from a State Hospital for the Insane; showing that he or she has attended said number of lectures; and has also attended medical and surgical cases in the hospital, and has had practical instruction in obstetrics outside of the hospital, under competent teachers, or instructors; or holds a certificate from a special hospital, showing not less than two years training and attendance upon the said number of lectures, and who shall also have taken a post graduate course, of not less than six months in a general hospital; or any nurse who can furnish proof of four consecutive years of experience in a hospital where systematic instruction in theory and practice has been given, even if the hospital did not issue diplomas at the time of his or her training, shall be eligible for license and registration as a trained nurse.

"Section 2.—That until Dec. 1st, 1903, any nurse who does not come within the above provisions, but who has had five years nursing experience, and who can furnish proof of good moral character and professional ability and who can pass the examination by the State Board, shall be eligible for license and registration.

"Section 3.—That it shall be the duty of the Superior Court Clerk of any County, on presentation of a certificate duly signed by three physicians, residing in North Carolina, certifying that the nurse applying for license is to their knowledge competent, having had necessary experience or training and is of good moral character, or who holds a certificate or diploma from a general hospital, together with a certificate of good moral character, to register the date of registration with the name and evidence of the applicant in a book to be kept for this purpose in his office marked 'Register of Trained Nurses,' and to issue to the applicant a certificate of each registration under the seal of the Superior Court of such county, Provided, such application be made within twelve months from the date of the ratification of this Act. The said Clerk shall be entitled to collect a fee of fifty cents for such certificate. After the expiration of twelve months from the ratification of this Act, upon presentation of a certificate from the State Board of Examiners, hereinafter provided for, it shall be the duty of the Superior Clerk of any County to register and issue a certificate to the applicant, as provided in Section 3.

"Section 4.—That there shall be established a State Board of Examiners of Trained Nurses, consisting of seven members, three physicians appointed by the President of the State Medical Society and four licensed nurses, belonging to the North Carolina State Nurses' Association, and appointed by their President, whose duty it shall be, after the expiration of twelve months from the ratification of this Act, to examine all applicants for license as trained nurses as to their qualifications and competency. Three members of this Board shall constitute a quorum and a majority of those present shall decide upon the qualification of the applicant. Candidates will be examined in elements of anatomy, physiology, medical, surgical, obstetrical and practical nursing, invalid cookery and household hygiene. The said Board shall be elected for three years and hold an annual meeting at time and place to be determined upon by the Board. In case of a vacancy from any cause, this Board or a quorum thereof, is empowered to fill such vacancy.

"Section 5.—Each application for examination shall be accompanied by One Dollar, and upon the issuing of a certificate, another dollar shall be paid, which fees shall go towards defraying the expenses of the Board. If the application, on examination, shall be found competent and qualified, the Board shall issue a certificate to that effect, which, upon being exhibited to the Clerk of the Superior Court of any County, shall entitle the applicant to license and registration as provided in Section 3.

"Section 6.—The State Board of Examiners of Nurses shall have the power to revoke any certificate or license issued in accordance with this Act by a majority vote of said Board for gross incompetency, dishonesty, habitual intemperance, or any act derogatory to the morals or standing of the profession of nursing as may be determined by the Board, but before any license or certificate shall be revoked, the holder thereof, shall be entitled to not less than twenty days notice of the charge against her or him, and of the time and place of hearing and determining of such charges, at which time and place she or he shall be entitled to be heard. Upon the revocation of any certificate or license it shall be the duty of the Secretary of the Board to strike the name of the holder thereof from the roll of registered nurses, and to notifiy the Superior Court Clerk of the County where the holder is registered, and upon receipt of notice the said Clerk shall cancel such registration. It shall further be the duty of the said Secretary of the Board to demand of the holder to surrender the certificate or license held by him or her.

"Section 7.—Any person who shall procure a license under this Act by means of any false and fraudulent representation or by the production of false certificate or testimonials, or who shall refuse to surrender for cancellation a certificate of registration or license which shall be revoked under the provisions of Sec. 6, shall be guilty of misdemeanor.

"Section 8.—In all appointments of nurses in hospitals under the control of the State, County or City, preference of employment in regard to future vacancies shall be given to registered nurses, provided that nothing herein contained shall be construed to interfere with the employment of pupil

nurses, and no pupil nurse who has had less than two years'
training shall be sent out to take charge of a private case.

"Section 9.—It shall not be lawful for any Hospital, Sanitarium or Training School in the State of North Carolina,
whether incorporated or otherwise, to issue diplomas, certificates or any other credentials certifying to the competency
of their pupils as trained or graduated nurses, unless they
have had the instruction, training and experience provided
for in Sec. 1 of this Act.

"Section 10.—This Act shall not be construed to affect or
apply to the gratuitous nursing of the sick by friends or
members of the family, or to any person nursing the sick
for hire who does not, in any way, assume to be a registered
or trained nurse.

"Section 11.—Every person who shall duly receive license
in accordance with the provisions of this Act, shall be known
and styled a 'Registered Trained Nurse,' and it shall be un-
lawful after twelve months from the passage of this Act, for
any person to practice professional nursing of the sick as
such without license in this State, or to advertise as, or assume the title of trained nurse, graduate nurse, or to use the
abbreviation of T.N., G.N., R.N. and R.G.N., or any other
words, letters or figures to indicate that the person using
the same is a trained, registered or graduate nurse.

"Section 12.—That this act shall be in force and effect
from and after its ratification."

The bill passed the House on January 28, 1903, without
difficulty. The press was loud in its praise for the legislators
who had aided the nurses in taking this progressive step. A
few days later it was learned that the bill had been held up
in the Senate and would be referred to the joint committee
on public health.

From the February, 1903, *News and Observer* of Raleigh,
North Carolina, the following is quoted: "Bill for Trained

Nurses Torn to Pieces. A substitute Recommended by Members of the Committee will be drawn and Its Passage Promised." The substitute bill which was passed is as follows:[1]

"Section 1.—That any nurse who may present to the clerk of the Superior Court in the State on or before December 31, 1903 a diploma from a reputable training school for nurses conducted in connection with a general hospital, public or private, in which medical, surgical, and obstetrical cases are treated, or in connection with one of the three State Hospitals for the insane, or who shall exhibit a certificate of attendance upon such training school for a period of not less than two years, or who shall present a certificate signed by three registered physicians stating that he or she has pursued as a business the vocation of a trained nurse for a period of no less than two years, and is in their judgment competent to practice the same, shall be entitled to registration without examinations, and shall be registered by the clerk of the Court in the manner hereinafter provided.

"Section 2.—On and after January 1, 1904 registration as a trained nurse shall be made by the Clerk of the Court solely upon the presentation to him of a license from the State Board of Examiners of Nurses as created and provided by this act.

"Section 3.—There shall be established a Board of Examiners of Nurses composed of five members, two physicians and three registered nurses to be elected by the Medical Society of the State of North Carolina and the North Carolina State Nurses' Association respectively, to be known by the title of 'The Board of Examiners of Trained Nurses of North Carolina.' Their term of office shall be three years. Three members, one of whom shall be a physician, shall constitute a quorum, and a majority of those present shall be a deciding vote. They shall each receive as compensation

[1] *Public Laws of North Carolina*, 1903, chap. ccclix, pp. 586-88.

for his or her services when engaged in the work of the Board four dollars a day and actual traveling and hotel expenses, the same to be paid out of money received from license issued, and in no case to be charged upon the Treasury of the State.

"Section 4.—The said Board of Examiners is authorized to elect such officers and frame such by-laws as may be necessary, and upon the occurrence of a vacancy is empowered to fill such vacancy for the unexpired term.

"Section 5.—At meetings it shall be their duty to examine all applicants for license as registered nurse, of good moral character, in the elements of anatomy and physiology, in medical, surgical, obstetrical and practical nursing, invalid cookery and household hygiene, and if on such examination they be found competent to grant each applicant a license authorizing her or him to register, as hereinafter provided, and to use the title 'Registered Nurse' signified by the letters R.N. The said Board of Examiners may in its discretion, issue license without examination to such applicants as shall furnish evidence of competency entirely satisfactory to them. Each applicant before receiving license, shall pay a fee of $5.00 which shall be used for defraying the expenses of the Board.

"Section 6.—The Clerk of the Superior Court of any county upon presentation to him of a license from the said Board of Examiners, shall register the date of registration with the name and residence of the holder thereof in a book to be kept in his office for this purpose and marked 'Register of Trained Nurses,' and shall issue to the applicant a certificate of such registration under the seal of the Superior Court of the County, upon the form furnished him as hereinafter provided, for which registration he shall be paid 50 cents by the applicant.

"Section 7.—It shall be the duty of the North Carolina State Nurses' Association to prescribe a proper form of the

Certificate required by this act, and to furnish the same in sufficient quantity suitably bound in a book and labeled 'Register of Trained Nurses' to the Clerk of the Court of each county in North Carolina.

"Section 8.—The said Board of Examiners shall have power after 20 days notice of the charges preferred and the time and place of meeting and after a full and fair hearing on the same by a majority vote of the whole Board, to revoke any license issued by them for gross incompetency, dishonesty, habitual intemperance, or any other act in the judgment of the Board derogatory to the morals or standing of the profession of nursing. Upon the revocation of a license or certificate the name of the holder thereof shall be stricken from the roll of registered nurses in the hands of the Secretary of the Board, and upon notification of such action by the said Secretary by the Clerk of the Court from his register.

"Section 9.—Any person procuring license under this act by false representation, or who shall refuse to surrender a license which has been revoked in the manner prescribed in Section 8, or who shall use the title 'R.N.' without first having obtained license to do so, shall be guilty of a misdemeanor, and upon conviction shall be fined not more than $50.00 or imprisoned not exceeding 30 days.

"Section 10.—Nothing in this act shall in any manner whatever curtail or abridge the right and privilege of any person to pursue the vocation of a nurse, whether trained or untrained, registered or not registered.

"Section 11.—This act shall be in force from and after its ratification."

Certain obscure points in the law of 1903 were clarified by the General Assembly in 1905:

"Section 5.—That after January 1, 1905, it shall be the duty of said Board of Examiners to meet not less frequently than once in every year, notice of which meeting shall be given in the public press."

Section 5[2] of the 1903 Nursing Law was amended at the 1907 session of the Legislature and was as follows: it required that in addition to being "of good moral character": (a) he or she must be more than 21 years of age; (b) have the equivalent of a high school education; and (c) have graduated from a training school connected with a general hospital or sanatorium where three years of training with a systematic course of instruction had been given in the hospital.

North Carolina was the first of the states to revise the Nursing Law, which was ratified on February 2, 1917. The revision is briefly outlined below:[3]

"That after June 1, 1917, no one shall represent herself or himself, or in any way assume to practice as a trained, graduate, licensed or registered nurse in North Carolina without obtaining a license through the Nurses' Examining Board." Nurses then practicing were to be permitted to register without examination from passage of the Act (Waiver: February 2, 1917, to June 1, 1917).

Section 1 (a) created a Board of Nurse Examiners composed, as originally, of five members, two physicians and three registered nurses, to be elected by the State Medical Society and the State Nurses' Association, respectively; (b) specified name of Board—the Board of Examiners of Trained Nurses of North Carolina; (c) specified the term of office of Board members—three years, terms to expire alternately— the Board to fill vacancies; (d) provided for inspector of training school; outlined qualifications, etc., of inspector, the inspector to be a registered nurse appointed annually by the State Nurses' Association, the duties and compensation to be fixed by the Board of Nurse Examiners and a report was to be made to the Board annually.

[2] *Ibid.*, 1907, chap. cccccxlii, p. 802.   [3] *Ibid.*, 1917, chap. xvii, p. 70.

Section 2 (a) specified number constituting a quorum (three: two to be nurses); (b) authorized the adoption of a seal; (c) authorized the adoption of by-laws and regulations for its own government and for the execution of the provisions of the Act; (d) named officers and provided for their election (president, secretary-treasurer, to be elected from the nurse members); (e) required bond of treasurer (amount of bond to be fixed by Board); (f) named compensation of Board members ($4.00 per day and actual expenses); (g) allowed salary to secretary-treasurer (amount to be fixed by Board—not to exceed $250 per year); (h) specified use of moneys received (to defray expenses of Board, to extend nursing education in the State).

Section 3 (a) specified frequency of examinations (not less frequent than once a year, or upon notice to secretary of ten or more applications); (b) required notice of examinations (notice to be given thirty days prior to examinations in one nursing journal and three daily State papers); (c) outlined duty of Board at such meeting (examination of graduate nurses applying for license to practice in North Carolina); (d) outlined requirements for eligibility to registration (must be proved to satisfaction of the Board that he or she: is 21 years of age; is of good moral character; has had one year of high school or its equivalent; has had three years' training in a general hospital giving a systematic course in theory and practice; or if trained in small, or special hospitals and sanatoria, to meet the above requirements by affiliations).

Section 4 (a) specified subjects in which examinations were held (anatomy, physiology, materia medica, dietetics, hygiene, elementary bacteriology, obstetrical, medical and surgical nursing, nursing of children, contagious diseases and ethics of nursing, and such other subjects as may be prescribed by the examining Board); (b) authorized granting of license, and use of title "Registered Nurse," "R.N."

(if applicant is found competent); (c) named a registration fee, ten dollars.

Section 5 provided for issuing license without examination to nurses registered in other states, said states to maintain equivalent standards of registration requirements.

Section 6 required nurses to register (all "trained," "graduate," "licensed," or "registered" nurses must obtain license from the Nurses' Examining Board before practicing in the State).

Section 7 specified the Act was not to affect gratuitous nursing by friends or members of the family; nurses sent into homes for hire by hospitals; nurses not representing themselves or assuming to practice as "trained," "graduate," "licensed," or "registered" nurses.

Section 8 required registration of certificate with the clerk of the Superior Court (clerk's fee fixed at fifty cents).

Section 9 (a) provided for revocation of license (upon conviction of gross incompetency, dishonesty, intemperance, or any act derogatory to the morals or standing of the profession, no license to be revoked except upon charges preferred, the accused to be furnished with written copy of such charges and given not less than twenty days' notice of time and place of hearing, the Board to accord a full and fair hearing); (b) provided for punishment for procuring license by false representation, or refusal to surrender a license which has been revoked, and named a penalty of fifty dollars or imprisonment not to exceed thirty days.

The amendment of 1919 was enacted to encourage better-educated women to enter the profession and also to increase the number of nurses to meet the postwar needs of the State.[4] This amendment provided "that training schools for nurses may give such credit for college work, on the three years' course as they may deem wise, such credit not to total more than one year for any one person."

[4] *Ibid.,* 1919, chap. cx, pp. 647-50.

The Nursing Law was again revised in 1925. The bill met with little or no opposition and was ratified on February 28, 1925. It was, briefly, as follows:[5]

Section 2 (a) created a Board of Nurse Examiners, composed, as originally, of five members: three nurses elected by the North Carolina State Nurses' Association, and one representative from the North Carolina Medical Society and one from the North Carolina Hospital Association; (b) specified the title of the Board—the Board of Nurse Examiners of North Carolina; (c) specified term of office of the Board members (three years or until successor qualified); (d) provided for filling vacancies on the Board (vacancy for unexpired term to be filled by the Board); (e) empowered the Board to prescribe regulations governing applicants for license, etc. (with approval of Standardization Board).

Section 3 (a) created a joint committee on Standardization, composed of three members appointed from the North Carolina State Nurses' Association, and three members from the North Carolina State Hospital Association; (b) specified term of office of members (three years or until successor qualified); (c) outlined duties of Standardization Board (to advise with the Board of Nurse Examiners in adoption of regulations governing applicants for license and standardization of schools of nursing; to classify schools of nursing, with the assent of the Board of Nurse Examiners; to prescribe rules and regulations for such classifications).

Section 4 provided for the appointment of an educational director of schools of nursing, and specified qualifications, duties, etc. (to be a registered nurse appointed annually by the North Carolina State Nurses' Association, to report annually to the Board of Nurse Examiners and the North Carolina State Hospital Association, the duties and compensation to be fixed by the Board of Nurse Examiners and Standardization Board).

[5] *Ibid.,* 1925, chap. lxxxvii, pp. 92-96.

Section 5 (a) specified number constituting a quorum (three: two nurses); (b) authorized the adoption of a seal; (c) authorized adoption of by-laws and regulations for its own government (the Board to frame by-laws and regulations for its own government and for execution of provisions of the Act); (d) provided for the election of officers (president, secretary-treasurer, to be elected from its nurse members); (e) required bond of treasurer (the amount of the bond to be fixed in by-laws and the premium thereof paid by the Board); (f) provided for compensation of Board members (compensation to be fixed by the Board); (g) provided for salary of secretary-treasurer (amount of salary to be fixed by the Board, salaries and expenses to be paid from fees received); (h) authorized use of money (all money in excess of allowance and expenses to be used for extending nursing education in the State).

Section 6 (a) specified frequency of meetings (not less frequently than once annually, or any time ten or more applicants notify the secretary-treasurer that they desire an examination); (b) required notice of examinations (notice to be given thirty days prior to examinations, in one nursing journal and three daily State papers); (c) outlined requirements for eligibility of those applying for license (21 years of age; of good moral character; one year of high school education or its equivalent and three years' training in a general hospital, meeting minimum requirements of the American Nurses' Association in effect at the time of the application; or, training in a small or special hospital or sanatorium meeting aforesaid requirements by affiliation with one or more schools of nursing).

Section 7 (a) specified subjects in which examinations were to be held (anatomy and physiology, materia medica, dietetics, hygiene and elementary bacteriology, obstetrical, medical, and surgical nursing, nursing of children, contagious diseases, and such other subjects as may be prescribed by the Examining Board); (b) authorized granting of license, and use of title "Registered Nurse," "R.N." (to those found competent), such nurses entitled to use "Registered Nurse," "R.N."; (c) fixed fee for registration by examination (ten dollars).

Section 8 (a) authorized granting of license without examination (to nurses registered in other states provided said states maintain equivalent standards of registration requirements, or to applicant registered in other states who possess qualifications at least equal to those required by the State of North Carolina); (b) fixed fee for registration without examination (twenty-five dollars).

Section 9 required nurses to register (all "trained," "graduate," "licensed," or "registered" nurses to obtain license from the Board of Nurse Examiners before practicing their profession in North Carolina).

Section 10 designated those not affected by the Act (the gratuitous nursing of friends or members of family; student nurses sent into homes by hospitals for hire; or persons who do not assume to practice as "trained," "graduate," "licensed," or "registered" nurses).

Section 10½ authorized rules of comity (the Board to make rules allowing registered nurses from other states to do temporary nursing in the State).

Section 11 required registration of license (nurses holding license from the North Carolina Board of Nurse Examiners to have it registered with a clerk of the Superior Court within twelve months after it is issued, the clerk's fee being fixed at fifty cents).

Section 12 (a) provided for revocation of license (upon conviction of gross incompetency, dishonesty, intemperance, or any acts derogatory to the morals or standing of the profession, no license to be revoked except upon charges preferred, the accused to be furnished with a written copy of such charges and given not less than twenty days' notice of time and place of hearing, the Board to accord a full and fair hearing); (b) required that the name be stricken from the roll upon revocation of license (secretary of the Board of Nurse Examiners and clerk of Superior Court to remove same from roll of registered nurses upon notice that license has been revoked).

Section 13 provided for prosecution for procuring license by false representation or refusal to surrender license which has been revoked, and named the penalty—a fine of not more than fifty dollars or imprisonment not to exceed thirty days.

A bill to amend the law was introduced in 1931 and ratified in February of the same year. The changes were, briefly, as follows:[6]

The name of the Board was changed to North Carolina Board of Nurse Examiners.

Section 3 provided for the Standardization Board to advise with the Board of Nurse Examiners in the adoption of regulations governing the education of nurses and to have power to establish standards and provide minimum requirements for the conduct of schools of nursing.

Section 6 (a) required that the applicant for registration be a high school graduate or have equivalent credits; (b) required that applicants be graduates of schools of nursing connected with general hospitals giving a three years' course of practical and theoretical instructions, said hospital to meet the minimum requirements and standards set up by the Committee on Standardization.

Section 10 designated those not affected by the Act (those engaged in the gratuitous nursing of the sick by friends or members of the family).

The Amendment of 1931 was substituted for a defeated bill and changed Section 3 of the Amendment of 1931 as follows:[7]

[6] *Ibid.,* 1931, chap. lvi, pp. 57-58.   [7] *Ibid.,* 1933, chap. cciii, p. 230.

"A joint committee on standardization, consisting of three members appointed from the North Carolina State Nurses' Association and four members from the North Carolina State Hospital Association whose members shall serve for a term of three years, or until their successors are elected, is hereby created. The joint committee on standardization shall advise with the Board of Nurse Examiners herein created in the adoption of regulations governing the education of nurses, and shall jointly with the North Carolina Board of Nurse Examiners have power to establish standards and provide minimum requirements for the conduct of schools of nursing of which applicants for examination for nurse's license under this chapter must be graduates before taking such examination."

Other legislation affecting nurses was sponsored by lay people, in which nurses took no part.

An act in 1915 provided for the establishment of a training school for nurses at the North Carolina State Tuberculosis Sanatorium.[8]

In 1915 a bill was passed in the legislature requiring public and private hospitals, sanatoriums, etc., in North Carolina, where colored patients were admitted for treatment and where nurses were employed, to employ colored nurses for the care of such colored patients. This Act was repealed in 1925.[9]

[8] *Consolidated Statutes of North Carolina*, 1919, chap. cx, p. 650.
[9] *Ibid.*, p. 651.

See Secretary's Book. P. 7.

Treasurers Book.

Board of Examiner of Trained Nurses
of North Carolina.

Money received from the first
applicants to before the Board
at its first meeting
Raleigh, N.C. May 24 & 25, 1904

Miss Hattie Lowry	5.00		
" Ida Thompson	5.00		
" Edith Redwine	5.00		
" Julia Stinson	5.00		
" Dora Hawkins	5.00		
June 6th 1904 Expenditures			
To Seeman Printery		12	50
Stamps		2	00
Stationary for Examination		1	50
July 24 Deposited Fidelity Bank		9	00
	$25.00	25	50

Mary L. Wyche

Page from Secretary-Treasurer's Book showing receipts and disbursements of the first State Board Examination, Raleigh, 1904

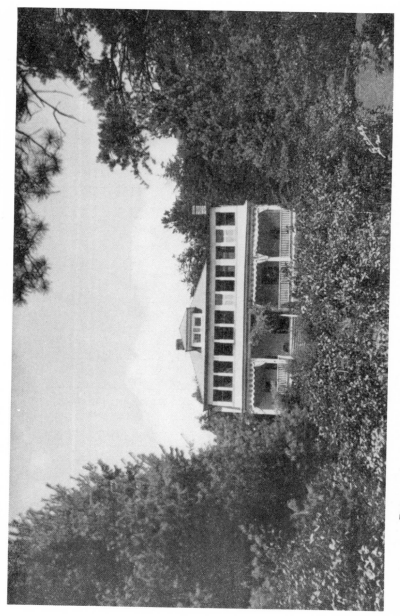

Dunnwyche, Mountain Home for Nurses, named for Miss Dunn and Miss Wyche

CHAPTER VIII

DUNNWYCHE

AND

THE NURSES' RELIEF FUND

THE MOVEMENT looking to the establishment of a home for the sick and disabled nurses conceived by Birdie Dunn of Raleigh was first proposed at the annual convention of the State Nurses' Association held in Greensboro in 1911. At that time the sum of three hundred and fifty dollars was pledged and fifty actually contributed. One year later something like seventeen hundred dollars was in hand with pledges for several hundred more. The site of two acres was contributed by Cragmont Sanatorium Company, through the kindly interest of Dr. I. J. Archer of Cragmont, and the Royal League—two neighboring sanatoriums situated two and one-half miles from Black Mountain. Dr. Archer generously gave professional services to the nurses. The home was primarily built for tubercular nurses from North Carolina where refined surroundings and moderate cost of living might be obtained.

The committee on ways and means for this undertaking had the courage to give the contract for the house, borrowing the needed amount to let the work go forward. The local associations and other nurses worked with the committee in splendid team work for the realization of their dreams. The Asheville Nurses' Association contributed one hundred dollars from a Christmas sale of dolls dressed as pupil nurses. Charlotte had tag day, bringing in three hundred and sixty dollars. Each group of nurses used whatever plan seemed best for raising money; somehow the money was raised and debts paid. Funds for the erection and support of Dunnwyche came as gifts of love from the nurses and their friends. With the gift often came a letter saying, "We count it a privilege to help in so noble an undertaking." At the meeting of the State Nurses' Association in 1910 a relief fund was created by increasing the annual dues one dollar. This was later used by Dunnwyche for improvements and current expenses.

In May, 1913, just two years after the building was started, it was formally turned over to the State Nurses' Association for guests. Some of the rooms were not completely furnished, but the patients who were taken in made the best of existing conditions.

The North Carolina State Nurses' Association met in Asheville in 1913 and one day was set apart to visit the Home, only fourteen miles away. The creation for which anxious hearts and hands had striven was viewed with pride. It was on this visit that the name "Dunnwyche" was suggested. The Home was soon after that christened "Dunnwyche" for Birdie Dunn and Mary Lewis Wyche. The name was chosen as an expression of appreciation of Miss Dunn's untiring efforts in building, furnishing, and directing the affairs of the Home, and of recognition of Miss Wyche's services to the State as organizer of the North Carolina State Nurses' Association, and as leader in the campaign for State registration. These two nurses gave from five to eight months of their time to the adjustment and management of Dunnwyche during its first year. Their positions as president and secretary-treasurer of the Board of Directors kept them in constant touch with the Home.

One year after it was completed, the original debt was cancelled. A furnace, electric lights, and increased sleeping porch space were the most urgent needs. For these improvements a new debt was contracted and disposed of in two years. Water from a spring near-by was a luxury from the first. This two-story building with all modern conveniences, beautifully situated on the mountain side, seemed ideal for its purpose.

Dunnwyche was governed by a Board of Directors, each local association electing one of its members to serve on this Board. Each of the seven associations furnished a room, bearing its name as indicated by a plate on the door, and made an annual donation of ten dollars for replenishing the linen. Many beautiful gifts of handiwork and ornaments were sent by the nurses and their friends and these helped to make it more homelike.

The patients were happy and optimistic. For entertainment they had card parties, automobile trips, and visits of friends and relatives—all of which helped to break the monotony of "taking the cure." There was a large living room with piano and victrola, an attractive dining room, and cosy little bedrooms off the well-arranged sleeping porch. The wonderful and soul-inspiring views of the valley and mountain range with its ever-changing panorama of the skies brought hope and cheer to those in search of health.

After America's entrance into the World War, when nurses and all other workers were diverted to new, and what seemed to them, more vital fields, Dunnwyche became a war victim.

A copy of the minutes of the Dunnwyche Board of Directors explains its fate:

"June 5, 1919.—Miss Dunn, secretary-treasurer of the Dunnwyche Board of Directors, read a report of the meeting of the directors held Wednesday afternoon. The report showed Dunnwyche in good financial condition; but after a careful consideration of the matter from every side the Board deemed it wise to advise the sale of Dunnwyche, owing to the continued increase of the cost of maintenance, the high cost of fuel and food brought about by war conditions, and also the question of suitable help to keep the house open. The demand for labor in the Government Hospital in the vicinity made it almost impossible to secure help. The Board thought the amount of energy expended too great for the amount of good accomplished in these strenuous times. It was suggested that the power of attorney be given Miss Wyche and Miss Dunn to dispose of Dunnwyche and to invest the money in Liberty Bonds; the interest accruing to be used for the benefit of nurses in ill health; the principal to be kept intact, hoping some day it might be possible for us to have a small cottage for our nurses at the State Sanatorium.

"A nurse from each local association in the State was asked to express an opinion. They unanimously agreed with the Board of Directors. Then the members of the Association voted to accept the recommendation of the Dunnwyche Board. A feeling of deep sadness prevailed and many tears were shed in the audience, as Dunnwyche meant so much to us. We felt that it had accomplished a great work, but as conditions existed in this time of the great World War, we could not let sentiment prevent our advising an act that we deemed best and thus making more money available for relief work.

(signed)   BIRDIE DUNN
Secretary-Treasurer"

Miss Dunn says, "But for the economic upheaval incident to war, Dunnwyche might have had many more years of usefulness. The disappointment connected with my dream of a permanent home for sick nurses would be insupportable did we not have some tangible remnant left, which may be added to from year to year and which, even now, may ease many a mind from the harrowing thought of illness and an accumulated debt."

Dunnwyche was greatly beloved by many nurses. A number have been restored to normal living and still others have been grateful for that last abiding place. So, after all, the work has not been in vain. Miss Dunn says, "Not that I would have it back—for I feel that there is too much work along preventive lines—and then it is still living in another form—'a loan for sick nurses.'"

A permanent State Relief Fund was established by investing the money received from the sale of Dunnwyche in United States Bonds. It has steadily increased over a period of twenty-five years by the payment of one dollar per capita by the members of the North Carolina State Nurses' Association. When the National Relief Fund was dissolved in 1932, North Carolina received her pro rata share which was added to the original investment. The by-laws specify that only the interest can be used for relief. By wise investment and careful distribution, the Fund has increased enough to enable the committee to aid many nurses who would otherwise have been in need.

Any nurse desiring relief must make application on blanks supplied for that purpose by the State Relief Fund chairman, and must have been a member of the North Carolina State Nurses' Association for five years preceding her illness. The amount given to each individual is left to the discretion of the committee.

The nurses who have served as chairmen of the Relief Fund and who have given much of their valuable time to keep this Fund intact are Birdie Dunn of Raleigh, E. A. Kelley of Fayetteville, Columbia Munds of Wilmington, and Jessie McLean of Greensboro.

CHAPTER IX

PUBLIC HEALTH NURSING

THE NORTH CAROLINA STATE BOARD OF HEALTH

THE ORGANIZATION of state boards of health was the direct result of the typhoid epidemics of the seventies which swept the country. The necessity of some organized effort for public health work was called to the attention of the people by a woman in Massachusetts.

North Carolina was the twelfth state to introduce legislation for the establishment of a state board of health. Through the untiring efforts of Dr. Thomas Fanning Wood of Wilmington, the Legislature passed a law on February 12, 1877, making the North Carolina Medical Society, which had been organized in 1849, the North Carolina State Board of Health. The sum of $100 annually was placed at the disposal of this organization to defray expenses. Combining these two organizations soon proved to be an unsatisfactory arrangement and the Legislature of 1879 passed a new law which put the State Board of Health on a separate and permanent basis with a financial appropriation of $200 annually.

The personnel is now composed of nine members, serving a term of four years each. Five members are appointed by the governor and four by the State Medical Society. Dr. Wood was the first secretary-treasurer and served in that capacity until his death, August 22, 1892. The appropriation made by the Legislature was inadequate from the beginning and Dr. Wood often used his personal funds to carry on the work.

Dr. Richard Henry Lewis of Raleigh was elected secretary of the State Board of Health in 1892 to succeed Dr. Wood. He held that office until 1909, and during this time the financial appropriation was raised to four thousand dollars a year, a meager sum for the scope of work which was done under Dr. Lewis' administration. Dr. Watson S. Rankin succeeded Dr. Lewis as secretary in 1909.

The activities of the State Board of Health are organized under nine divisions as follows: Administrative, Preventive Medicine and Hygiene, Sanitary Engineering, Oral Hygiene, State Laboratory of Hygiene, Epidemiology, Vital Statistics, County Health Work, and Industrial Hygiene.

The division of Preventive Medicine and Hygiene is of vital interest to nurses. They are the pioneers in this branch of the work. Subdivisions of this department include School Health Supervision, National and Child Health Service, and Health Education.

In 1915 Dr. George M. Cooper of Clinton was appointed director of the Bureau of Rural Sanitation on the executive staff of the State Board of Health. He launched a program for the improvement of rural sanitation which was badly needed in all small towns and counties. During the summer months his efforts were directed to the eradication of typhoid fever. He also realized the need for a system of medical inspection of school children in the elementary grades. This he arranged to have done during the school term with funds which were obtained from county authorities, private subscriptions, and social agencies. Three physicians, assisted by several senior medical students, were assigned this work the first year. By the end of 1916 Dr. Cooper, realizing that his efforts would be futile unless a follow-up system could be provided, made a survey which disclosed that good advice had been given but very little of it had been heeded by the parents of the school children.

The Legislature of 1917 passed a law requiring periodic examination of the school child every three years but no provision was made for the salary of the physician. The county authorities were called upon to supply funds for the doctors' salaries; this produced complications. Enough good had been accomplished, however, to prove that lasting benefits were being derived from the movement. This fact encouraged Dr. Cooper to feel that he could make better plans for the future. The great need was for a systematized follow-up program which could be controlled by the director and financed by the State Board of Health.

Dr. Cooper had the privilege of writing the law, enacted by the Legislature in 1919, providing for periodic inspection of school children and an appropriation for the salaries of the physicians. The term "Agent" inserted into the law applied to physicians, dentists, teachers, and nurses. It was Dr. Cooper's idea to appoint capable, well-trained graduate nurses for the work of school inspection. He realized that they could reach mothers and teachers and would coöperate with physicians in private practice.

The first nurses appointed to carry out this program of School Health Work were Cleone E. Hobbs of Clinton, Birdie Dunn of Raleigh, Cora E. Beam of Fallstone, Kate Livingstone[1] of Wagram, Flora Ray of Sanford, and Mrs. H. P. Guffy of Statesville. Since that time two other nurses, Mrs. Margaret Sloan and Mrs. Mozelle Hendrix, have been added to the personnel. These nurses have worked in practically every county in the State. The first six nurses have been with the State Board of Health over a period of eighteen years. Their duties consist of weighing and measuring each child, testing the vision and hearing, examining the teeth and throat, taking the family history and the

[1] Kate Livingstone died May 26, 1938.

child's history relative to what immunization has been given and what communicable diseases the child has had. This service is available to all white and negro school children.

The work of this group of nurses has been phenomenal in many respects. In the beginning only twenty counties had either a city or county health department, but due to their pioneer work the State now has sixty-five county and city health departments. The nurses go to the remaining counties biennially to make inspections. The success which has been met is largely due to the splendid efforts of the first six nurses. "They have traveled on foot, horseback, on rafts, by boat, tram cars, ox-carts—any way to reach the 'forgotten' child."

In 1919 the division of Infant Hygiene, financed jointly by the American Red Cross and the State Board of Health, appointed Miss M. Ehrenfeld as director of the department. Katherine Myers was appointed her assistant. Miss Ehrenfeld continued in this capacity for two years, carrying on a general program of public health. Her attention was focused on the welfare of maternity patients and the instruction of midwives. During a reorganization period in 1922 Miss Ehrenfeld was appointed health director of District No. 4. Miss Myers was retained as supervising nurse for the Red Cross with headquarters at the State Board of Health. The appointment of field nurses made it possible for this department to enlarge its scope of work. It now includes regular inspection of school children and classes for midwives during the summer months. Literature pertaining to all phases of maternity and child health and training are distributed to the public upon request by the Department of Preventive Medicine and Hygiene.

Following the inspection of the school child for defects arose the problem of the correction of these defects. Dr. Cooper instituted two experiments; namely, teaching oral hygiene, and organizing tonsil and adenoid clinics. Six dentists gave demonstrations throughout the counties, using portable equipment to teach oral hygiene to the school child. The experiment proved beneficial and now there are about twenty-five dentists doing this type of work in North Carolina.

The nurses were instrumental in organizing the tonsil and adenoid clinics under the direction of eye, ear, nose, and throat specialists. These physicians had agreed to perform the operations for a stipulated fee and to render service gratis for patients who could not afford any fee. Instead of a five-year program, as first outlined by Dr. Cooper, this service was conducted over a period of twelve years.

According to information furnished by the North Carolina State Board of Health, there are now one hundred and ninety-one public health nurses employed in the state, county, and city health departments. Two are in the State Health Department, ten are supervising nurses, one hundred and twenty-five are staff nurses (white), and thirty are staff nurses (Negro), distributed in fifty-four counties and five city health departments.

City and County Health Work

The early records of St. Peter's Hospital, Charlotte; St. John's, Raleigh; Flower Mission, Asheville; and the Twin-City Hospital, Winston-Salem, show that they started what was known then as "community" or "visiting" nursing among the sick poor of the towns. A student nurse was designated to visit and care for them in their homes under the direction of a physician. The funds and supplies for this branch of work were furnished by the hospital or, in some cases, by the town. This practice was discontinued when it became apparent that it was the work of the community rather than the hospital.

The next movement to care for charity patients was made by the various benevolent societies, civic organizations, and public-spirited citizens. They saw the need for tuberculosis control, school-child inspection, and a generalized nursing service. The salaries of the first nurses were paid by them and they were the promoters of the well-organized Public Health Service which prevails in North Carolina today. The Red Cross sent a number of graduate nurses into the State between May 1, 1915, and April, 1935. They were stationed in fifty-two counties and had a large part in developing the Public Health Service.

Wilmington has the distinction of having the first graduate nurse for visiting among the sick poor. In 1904 Amelia Lawrison was employed to do this work, her salary being paid by a small group of citizens. In 1907 the Ministering Circles of the King's Daughters assumed the responsibility of the visiting nurse and in 1917 employed a second nurse.

The Wayside Workers of the Home Moravian Church secured the services of a practical nurse to work among the people of Salem. She was replaced in 1911 by a registered nurse, Percy Powers, a graduate of St. Luke's Hospital, Bethlehem, Pennsylvania. She was also sent into East and West Salem schools to do inspection and follow-up work among the school children. This is the first record of school nursing in the State. Special permission was granted the Wayside Workers to get this branch of the work started.

When Miss Powers resigned in 1917 to become supervisor of nurses with the City Health Department of Winston-Salem, the Wayside Workers agreed to contribute ninety dollars per month toward the salary of a nurse connected with the health department, if she were allowed to continue the work started by Miss Powers. This arrangement prevailed over a period of four and one-half years. After that time the City Health Department took over school nursing.

In 1910 Asheville had a dispensary in connection with one of the hospitals and a graduate nurse, Jane Brown, was placed in charge of it to do general follow-up work and bedside nursing.

By 1911 there was considerable growth in the number of persons employed to do this type of nursing. Greensboro had a tuberculosis worker, paid from the fund derived from the sale of Christmas Seals; the Associated Charities of Raleigh employed a visiting nurse. They are still responsible for the salaries of two nurses, one white and one Negro.

Mrs. Clyde Dickson was employed in Durham in 1912 by the City and County Health Department to do visiting nursing. She is apparently the first nurse to engage in this work directly under the supervision of the health department. In 1915 Mrs. Emily Jenkins Pickard, a graduate of Watts Hospital, Durham, was appointed by the City School Board to start school nursing.

By this time the demands were greater and better organization was needed to develop a good public health program. Public health has been defined as "the art and science of preventing disease, prolonging life, and promoting physical and mental efficiency through organized community efforts." There was a definite need for closer coöperation with the medical agencies to produce the best results.

In this short history of nursing only a condensed report of the reorganization of some of the county and city health departments can be given.

Greensboro, in Guilford County, has the distinction of having established the first County Health Department in the United States on June 1, 1911. In 1918 Mary Horry was employed to do Infant Relief Work. Mrs. Blanche T. Lambe became the first school nurse in 1919. The department grew slowly and in 1925 the Greensboro Nursing Council was formed. It was comprised of all health organizations; namely, City School Board, City Health Department, County School Board, and the Metropolitan Life Insurance Company. Ten nurses were employed with Mrs. Lambe as the first supervising nurse. In 1926 Mrs. Lambe resigned and was succeeded by Mrs. Myrtle F. Robertson.

In 1937 the Greensboro Nursing Council had in the department eleven nurses, one part-time clerk, and a supervising nurse, Mrs. Lewis Raulston.

In 1909 the General Assembly of North Carolina provided that the Board of Aldermen of the city of Durham should appoint a board of health to be known as a "City Board of Health." It was to be composed of five members, two of which were physicians in good standing in the Durham County Medical Society. Dr. N. M. Johnson was the first health officer. In 1913 another act was passed which gave Durham a combined city and county board of health, financed jointly by the city and county. From this small beginning has grown a well-organized department with a full-time health officer and an active nursing staff.

Dr. J. J. Kinyoun of the United States Public Health Service, Washington, D. C., was sent to Winston-Salem in 1916 to act in an advisory capacity during a serious scarlet-fever epidemic. As a result of his work the City Health Department was organized in April, 1916. Mrs. Sallie Hardister Cook (white) and Girlie Jones Strickland (Negro) were employed for school and contagious work.

In 1917 Dr. R. L. Carlton of Winston-Salem was appointed whole-time health officer and Percy Powers became supervising nurse. Both Dr. Carlton and Miss Powers are still in office. The department is financed by the city of Winston-Salem and by funds derived from the sale of Christmas Seals. A staff of graduate nurses is composed of the supervisor, five school nurses (white), two school nurses (Negro), one special tuberculosis worker (white), and one special tuberculosis worker (Negro).

In October, 1917, Dr. C. C. Hudson took charge of the health work in Charlotte and found two nurses doing general bedside nursing. Their salaries were paid by the Metropolitan Life Insurance Company and the Young Men's Benevolent Society of the Second Presbyterian Church. A short time later, Stella Tylski of the American Red Cross Nursing Service, Washington, D. C., enlarged the organization by adding four field workers. She was also instrumental in getting two of the mills to add two nurses for bedside nursing and tuberculosis work among their employees. The Red Cross unit was withdrawn gradually, so that the department was not depleted at any time. In 1919 Dr. Hudson was successful in organizing the Charlotte Coöperative Nursing Association with Miss G. E. Reynolds as supervising nurse. Her salary was paid by the City Health Department and a number of civic organizations contributed to the general support of the organization.

In 1921 Charlotte had a generalized and specialized nursing service with Dr. W. A. McPhaul as health officer. The salary of the personnel was paid by lay people and official agencies. Seventeen nurses were employed.

In 1934 the Metropolitan Life Insurance Company's contract was not renewed, their service being done by nurses employed by the company.

In 1934 school nursing under the Board of Education was discontinued but resumed in September, 1935, under the City Health Department with Clara Ross, director of nursing, and Mrs. Martha T. Wright, supervisor of school health work. In 1937 the staff consisted of eighteen nurses doing a generalized work in that many districts, their salaries being paid by the Charlotte Coöperative Nursing Association and other agencies.

After a conference called by Dr. Charles E. Low, health officer, between representatives of the Board of Health, Red Cross, and Ministering Circle of the King's Daughters, the Wilmington Public Health Nursing Association was organized in 1918 with a supervising nurse and four staff nurses to work directly under the health officer. Columbia Munds was elected supervising nurse. She is still serving in that capacity. Since that time the Board of Health has employed a county nurse, the Jewish Women's Federated Charities contributed the salary for another city nurse, and two Negro nurses are paid by other special agencies.

In 1937 the staff consisted of a supervisor, four city staff nurses (white), two city staff nurses (Negro), two county nurses. The Social Security funds have made it possible to have these additional nurses.

The Public Health Department for the city and county was established in Raleigh in 1918 under the direction of Dr. C. E. Waller of the United States Health Service. A staff of six nurses was employed. The law provided that a physician and nurse should serve on the Board. Mrs. C. B. Barbee was appointed a nurse member in 1918 and is still serving. Flora R. Wakefield, of Lenoir, was appointed supervising nurse of the Wake County Health Department, August, 1937.

The Asheville Association for Public Health Nursing was organized from representatives of lay and official agencies in 1919. The city was divided into three districts with one nurse for each district. By 1923 the number of nurses had increased to six. The salaries of the nurses were being paid by funds derived from the Associated Charities, fees collected from Metropolitan Life Insurance policyholders, and the City School Board. This same year the work was taken over by the city commissioners and has been under their direction since that time.

CHAPTER X

THE ESTABLISHMENT OF NEGRO HOSPITALS AND THE PROGRESS OF NEGRO NURSES

THE NEGROES recognized the need for the establishment of separate hospitals and schools for nurses as early as 1888. The idea was sponsored by churches, public-spirited citizens, and city governing boards. They have progressed with the times by enlarging their buildings, adding equipment, and graduating more nurses. Several of the schools for nurses are accredited by the North Carolina Board of Nurse Examiners.

The Negro graduate nurses organized a Negro Nurses' Association in 1920. One of the most influential nurses in the State is Carrie Early Broadfoot. A short résumé of the establishment of the most prominent hospitals, the organization of the Negro Nurses' Association, and the life of Carrie Early Broadfoot are worthy of space in *The History of Nursing in North Carolina.*

GOOD SAMARITAN HOSPITAL

The General Convention of the Episcopal Church, organizers of the Good Samaritan Hospital in Charlotte, made appeals for funds in 1881 but the cornerstone was not laid until 1888. It was built for the care of sick negroes and for a training school for their race. The bed capacity is sixty-two. The school is still in operation. They have six graduate nurses on the staff. Marion Bodie is superintendent of the hospital.

LEONARD HOSPITAL

The Leonard Hospital of Raleigh was established by the Medical Department of Shaw University in 1885 with a bed capacity of forty. It was the first hospital in the State which employed only graduate nurses. Annie Groves was the first superintendent of nurses. The hospital closed in 1914 because of insufficient funds.

ST. AGNES' HOSPITAL

St. Agnes' Hospital is a department of St. Augustine School, Raleigh, North Carolina, founded in 1867 for young Negro men and women.

During the General Convention of the Episcopal Church held in Minneapolis, Minnesota, in 1895, the wife of A. B. Hunter, principal of St. Augustine's School, told of the great need of a hospital in which the Negroes of Raleigh might get the proper care and attention. One man gave $600 toward such a hospital and another special gift increased the hospital fund to about $6,000.

After looking for a suitable building for a hospital, attention centered upon the former residence of Dr. Sutton on the school grounds. This building was enlarged and altered and on St. Luke's Day, October 18, 1896, St. Agnes' Hospital was formally opened. Work began that day. It was dedicated by the church, and has developed into one of the most important institutions in the church. It has a wide influence and is doing much to mold the future of the Negro race.

The school staff regarded it only as a makeshift. The one faucet in the kitchen supplied water for the entire house. Hot water for operating and bathing purposes was heated on the wood stove which was the only means of supplying heat for any part of the building. Ice was used only in an emergency. Colder water than the faucet supplied was brought from a spring by the nurses to bathe typhoid patients, "old-fashioned typhoid" lasting many weeks. Two small sterilizers of uncertain action formed a part of the operating room equipment. A probationer standing just outside the operating room handed in hot water and received buckets of waste water from the operating room.

There were no plumbing facilities, no screens, no electric lights, no gas for cooking or lighting—only oil lamps. For laundry equipment three ordinary wash tubs served, together with a big iron pot in the yard for boiling clothes, and a flatiron heater. "The office was reception room, Doctor's living room, dining room, surgeon's dressing room on operating days, and sometimes the morgue."

In 1900 Dr. Catherine P. Hayden was installed as resident physician and superintendent of nurses. Later Edna H. Wheeler came to look after the housekeeping and linen. Mrs. Hunter was superintendent and treasurer. At an earlier date a medical and surgical staff had been appointed, with Dr. Hubert A. Royster as chief surgeon. "These men were called on any hour of the day or night" and they came, "walking through . . . red mud up to and above their ankles in bad weather. These men still stand just as ready today to give themselves for any emergency and to respond in season and out of season."

St. Agnes' Hospital with approximately one hundred beds is now a modern and well-equipped hospital, meeting the requirements of the Standardization Board.

The first head nurse of St. Agnes' Hospital was Marie Louise Burgess, a graduate of the New England Hospital for Women in Boston. Though only two pupil nurses constituted the beginning of the "school," lectures and recitations were regularly held, and surgical operations were a scheduled part of the day from the first. In the early life of the school one and a half years was the period of training required; later the course was extended to three years, thus meeting the demands of the law. The first two graduates of the class of 1898 were Anna A. Groves and Effie Wortham. A report of 1938 shows that two hundred and fifty-seven nurses have graduated from the school. Mrs. Frances A. Worral is director of the school of nurses.

LINCOLN HOSPITAL

The Lincoln Hospital was organized in 1901 primarily for the care of Negroes in the vicinity of Durham. It is supported by taxes and is under city government. A training school was established in 1902 with Julia A. Latta as the first superintendent of nurses. The hospital and training school is now directed by Helen P. Carter.

THE COMMUNITY HOSPITAL

Assisted by a group of interested citizens in 1920, Dr. F. F. Burnett and Dr. John Kay of Wilmington established the Community Hospital, located on Seventh Street. The bed capacity was twenty-two but in 1933 it was increased to thirty-four. A school of nursing was incorporated in 1920 and discontinued in 1936. Twenty-two nurses were graduated during that time. Salome Taylor, a graduate of Lincoln Hospital, New York City, is the superintendent of the hospital.

NEGRO DIVISION OF THE STATE SANATORIUM

The Negro division of the State Sanatorium at Sanatorium was opened on October 1, 1923. It is an integral part of the State Sanatorium, having cared for a large number of tuberculous Negroes. The State provided a building for this division at a cost of two hundred and fifty thousand dollars. A training school for Negro nurses was organized in 1926 and two nurses, Claretta Redding of Franklinton and Mary Elliott of Tremont, were graduated in the first class, May 28, 1928. Carrie Early Broadfoot has been in charge of this division of the State Sanatorium since its beginning.

L. RICHARDSON MEMORIAL HOSPITAL

The L. Richardson Memorial Hospital of Greensboro, which opened May 18, 1927, was built for the care of sick Negroes. The movement for this hospital began in January, 1923, when a group of colored people, realizing the need for such an institution, met and formed the Greensboro Negro Association. A charter was secured and there were seventy-two charter members. An amendment was made later which provided for a Board of Directors consisting of an equal number of white and colored citizens.

The family of Mrs. L. Richardson of Greensboro made a donation of $50,000 and the family of Mrs. Emanuel Sternberger gave $10,000 for the equipment of the operating room and for an X-ray machine. Large donations from the Rosenwald and Duke funds made it possible for a nurses' home to be added in 1929. The hospital has a bed capacity of sixty-four with a daily average of thirty. The training school is under the direction of Geneva Sitrena Collins, a graduate of St. Agnes' Hospital, Raleigh. In 1930 they graduated the first class with seven members.

NEGRO NURSES' ASSOCIATIONS

In August, 1920, at a meeting of the National Association of Negro Graduate Nurses in Washington, D. C., a group of five nurses from North Carolina who were attending the meeting were called together by Carrie Early Broadfoot and discussed plans for organizing a state association. This group spent the following year in writing letters to other graduate nurses advising them of what had been accomplished and trying to get them interested in a state association. A call meeting was held in Winston-Salem in January, 1923, and a permanent organization was formed with Carrie Early Broadfoot as president. She served in this capacity until the State Association was incorporated under the laws of North Carolina in 1931.

The first state-wide meeting was held in Raleigh in 1923 with thirty-five nurses present. Annual meetings have been held since organization, and the membership is now approximately one hundred and fifty. The association is divided into three districts, with headquarters at Winston-Salem, Raleigh, and Fayetteville. Ruby F. Scarlette of Greensboro is president of the State Association.

CARRIE EARLY BROADFOOT

One of the most prominent members of the Negro Nurses' Association is Carrie Early Broadfoot of Virginia. She was educated in the public schools of Lynchburg. Left an orphan at the age of seventeen years, she was thrown on her own resources.

Her professional training was received in the Frederick Douglas Memorial Hospital in Philadelphia, Pennsylvania, where she was graduated at the head of her class. She engaged in private duty nursing in Philadelphia for eighteen months after her graduation, and for the following five years she was superintendent of nurses of the Frederick Douglass Memorial Hospital, Philadelphia. She has held several other executive positions, one of them being superintendent of nurses of St. Agnes' Hospital, Raleigh, for two years. Nurse Broadfoot has taken every advantage which presented itself to broaden her education. After her marriage she attended summer school in Fayetteville five consecutive years. She joined the Red Cross and was anxious to go overseas but instead was called to give her services in the influenza epidemic which was sweeping the country at that time.

She has held many responsible positions and has served as a state officer and on special committees, among which are the following: president, Negro State Nurses' Association; member of the Executive Board; and recording secretary of the National Association of Negro Nurses.

IN MEMORIAM

Death is the port where all may refuge find,
The end of labour, entry into rest.
—WILLIAM ALEXANDER, *Tragedy of Darius*

Alford, Annie Henrietta
(Mrs. S. G. Kinlaw)
*Alford, Jessie B.
Atwell, Mary Selena
Baker, Alice
Barker, Swannie
Barrs, Louise Loman
Batterham, Mary Rose
Baumberger, Fannie Eliza
Beach, Ada Erin
Bell, Celeste (Mrs. S. A. Stevens)
Boone, Harriet Anne
Bowers, Ruby Mae
Boyles, Ella Mae
Boyles, Ona Mae
Brady, Sara Sybil
Britt, Mary M.
(Mrs. Norman Grant)
Brown, Effie Olia
Brown, Ella Louise
(Mrs. Romus T. White)
Brown, Sara Ellen
Bullock, Lillian
Bullock, Lillian Burns
Burden, Margaret P.
Camp, Elizabeth
Campbell, Belle
Chapin, Elizabeth C.
(Mrs. Jack Prichard)
Clark, Mrs. Earl H.

Clark, Margaret
Cockran, Mrs. Daisy D.
Collins, Lucy Edith
Combs, Elizabeth
Cox, Carrie Lee
Coxe, Gertrude Jones
Cranford, Roxie Ludora
Crouch, Mary Katherine
Daniels, Maisie V.
Davids, Anna H.
Dearman, Lily Leigh
Detwiler, Mary Horning
Dhylentis, Mrs. Ruby Mangum
Dolphy, M. Louise
Donald, Genieve Lee
Dudley, Marinda Jane
Dula, Frances Webb
Dumas, Katherine C.
Eckles, Jane Ann
Edwards, Imo Lee
Farmer, Nina Lewis
Ferguson, Margaret B.
Fitzgerald, Zelda A.
Flora, Hannah
Foister, Mable Hortense
Frazier, Mary
Freeman, Lucia
Fulcher, Nettie Mae
(Mrs. Earl Dawson)

* Negro nurse.

Goswick, Martha
  (Mrs. Phillip Sims)
Graham, Allie
Greene, Dolly Emma
Hall, Sallie Ethel
Haltiwanger, Janet Sims
  (Mrs. David Johnson)
Hardaway, Annie G.
Harris, Mrs. Evelyn Spruce
Hartsell, Virginia
Hatfield, Mrs. Effie Ray
Hawkins, Annie M.
Hazelton, Sallie H.
Hemphill, Grace M.
Hendren, Carmine Marguerite
Hinson, Pauline E.
Holmes, Ethel Edith
Holmes, Maude
Holthouser, Ruby
Holton, Mary M.
  (Mrs. John Boney)
Hughes, Madeline K.
  (Mrs. Viall)
Hume, Jane
Humphries, Eugenia Frances
Insch, Annie M.
Irwin, Susan Verna
Israel, Mary Bertha
Jarvis, Sara E.
  (Mrs. All Heron)
Jessup, Claudia
  (Mrs. R. C. Perry)
Jones, Dixon Lidie
Josenhous, Charlotte Rose
Kelly, Sibbie A.
Kendall, Mary L.
Kendrick, Sara Adelia
Key, Christine E.
Kirby, Leah Mae
Klutz, Janet Craig

Kuykendall, Hallie L.
  (Mrs. A. V. Russell)
Langston, Marie Howell
  (Mrs. R. G. Watson)
Laurance, Mrs. Marion H.
Leech, Garfield
Lewis, Margaret T.
Lilly, Estelle V.
Lippard, Mary Elizabeth
Little, Jane
Livingston, Louise
  (Mrs. Rudolph Gerber)
Lofton, Mary
Long, Bertha
Lord, Athelia
Loving, Mrs. Allen Crews
Lyman, Kathryn
MacNichols, Caroline E.
Masten, Lydia Katherine
  (Mrs. J. Howard Barnes)
Mathews, Flora
Mauney, Catherine Perkins
McCluna, Matilda
McConnell, Mary
McCracken, Sara Emily
McIver, Kathleen (Mrs. Viall)
McLaughlin, Annie Bryce
  (Mrs. Beam)
McMulkin, Mary J.
McNeil, Flora Fletcher
Moody, Beulah F.
Morris, Annie
Mullen, Eloise Gertrude
Norton, Lonnie Dudley
Overby, Pattie E.
Owings, Kitty Burns
Palmer, Eva
Page, Lucy
Parker, Lucille Cameron
  (Mrs. Nash Penny)

Patterson, Lula Troy
Pepper, Hattie
Perkins, Etta Mae
Petteway, Gertrude Lillian
Phillips, Nell Allen
  (Mrs. W. B. Bush)
Pinner, Christie McRae
Pinyon, Sara Ann
Pinyon, Theresa
Plyler, Eleanor
Polk, Emma Lee
Pratt, Nannie
Price, Mrs. Julia R.
Ray, Beatrice Marie
Reveley, Annie Dade
Rhodes, Cora Lee
Robertson, Ada H.
Robertson, Margaret Reid
Robinson, Annabel
Rogers, Mary Ruth
  (Mrs. S. T. Ballard)
Rogers, Nora Rebecca
  (Mrs. Deering)
Rosser, Fairy
  (Mrs. Henry Steele)
Rothwell, Katherine
Royall, Frances (Mrs. Ross)
Saunders, Myrtle Iola
Sellers, Mary Louise
  (Mrs. J. B. Gordon)
Shook, Maggie
Shore, Bertie Bernice
Shroat, Annie Elizabeth
Simpson, Carrie Annie
Sisk, Lela
Smith, Ella Price

Smith, Loyselle
Smith, Marie Lovie
Smith, Viola G.
Sodini, Marie Elizabeth
  (Mrs. Angelo)
Spann, Matilda Erwin
  (Mrs. Marvin Turner)
Speight, Emma
Stapleford, Shelly Catherine
Stokes, Bertha Gray
Story, Samuel
Strickland, Selina Irene
Sutton, Mary
  (Mrs. George Autry)
Sykes, Nora Lee
*Taylor, Elina Dancy
*Teer, Daisy B.
Thompson, Lela Stamey
Tuten, Pearl Evelyn
Vanstory, Elizabeth
Walker, Charlotte Minchin
Walston, Bessie B.
Watson, Alice
Watson, Ellen S.
Webb, Mrs. Fannie M.
White, Martha Phylena
Williams, Lillian R.
Willis, Annie Belle
Woltz, Alice
Wood, Dianna
  (Mrs. Raymond Dean)
Wortham, Effie
  (Mrs. Wortham Lytle)
Wright, Elizabeth M.
Wyche, Mary Lewis
Yow, Annie (Mrs. Rucker)

* Negro nurse.

APPENDIX A

CHARTER MEMBERS OF NORTH CAROLINA STATE NURSES' ASSOCIATION*

Barrett, Raleigh
†Mary Rose Batterham, Asheville
Mary Battle, Asheville
†Annie Bell Bledsoe, Raleigh
Lizzie Blow, Raleigh
Iphigenia Bowen, Durham
Ella Case, Asheville
H. P. Clegg, Greensboro
†Jennie Coffin, Raleigh
Nannie Lou Crowson, Raleigh
Georgia Dalton, Winston-Salem
Anna Lee de Vane, Raleigh
Birdie Dunn, Raleigh
Hester Evans, Asheville
Anne Ferguson, Statesville
Lena L. Gilliland, Winston-Salem
Laura Grim, Asheville
Sophie Grimes, Raleigh
Selma A. Hayes, Raleigh
Eugenia Henderson, Winston-Salem
Z. B. Henderson, Morganton
Jennie Higgs, Raleigh

Rosa G. Hill, Raleigh
Cleone E. Hobbs, Greensboro
†Jane Hume, Arden
Maude Keith, Asheville
L. M. King, Raleigh
†Marion H. Laurance (Mrs.), Raleigh
Lena Mary Lee, Raleigh
†Athalia Lord, Asheville
Mary Martin, Winston-Salem
Adeline Orr, Asheville
Constance E. Pfohl, Winston-Salem
Mary D. Pittman, Raleigh
Belle Reece, Asheville
Mary Sheetz, Raleigh
†Emma S. Speight, Brinkleyville
Annie Sturgeon, Raleigh
Maude Truman, Raleigh
Elizabeth Walker, Statesville
Daisy Wallace, Raleigh
†E. May Williams, Davidson
†Mary Wyche, Raleigh

* Two names are missing.
† Deceased.

APPENDIX B

NORTH CAROLINA STATE NURSES' ASSOCIATION
1902-1938

Year	President	Secretary	Place
1902	Mary L. Wyche	Anna Lee de Vane	Raleigh
1903	Mary L. Wyche	Constance Pfohl	Asheville
1904	Mary L. Wyche	Constance Pfohl	Raleigh
1905	Mary L. Wyche	Constance Pfohl	Winston-Salem
1906	Mary L. Wyche	Constance Pfohl	Charlotte
1907	Mary L. Wyche	Constance Pfohl	Richmond, Va.
1908	Constance Pfohl	Mary Sheets	Durham
1909	Constance Pfohl	Mary Sheets	Wrightsville Beach
1910	Constance Pfohl	Mary Sheets	Asheville
1911	Constance Pfohl	Lois Toomer	Greensboro
1912	Constance Pfohl	Lois Toomer	Charlotte
1913	Constance Pfohl	Dorothy Hayden (Mrs.)	Asheville
1914	Cleone Hobbs	E. May Williams	Durham
1915	Cleone Hobbs	E. May Williams	Wilmington
1916	Cleone Hobbs	Dorothy Hayden (Mrs.)	Winston-Salem
1917	Eugenia Henderson	Dorothy Hayden (Mrs.)	Fayetteville
1918	Eugenia Henderson	Blanche Stafford	Kinston
1919	Eugenia Henderson	Blanche Stafford	Asheville
1920	Blanche Stafford	Carolyn Miller	Charlotte
1921	Dorothy Hayden (Mrs.)	Carolyn Miller	Wilmington
1922	Dorothy Hayden (Mrs.)	Harriet Lesowski	Greensboro
1923	Pearl Weaver	Athalia Lord	Raleigh

1924	Blanche Stafford	Edna Heinzerling	Winston-Salem
1925	Blanche Stafford	Edna Heinzerling	Asheville
1926	Columbia Munds	Bessie Powell	Goldsboro
1927	Columbia Munds	Bessie Powell	Charlotte
1928	Mary P. Laxton	Dorothy Wallace	Durham
1929	Mary P. Laxton	Dorothy Wallace	Wrightsville Beach
1930	E. A. Kelley	Leckie Ballard	Greensboro
1931	E. A. Kelley	Martha C. Newman	Blue Ridge
1932	Hettie Reinhardt	Flora Wakefield	Raleigh
1933	Hettie Reinhardt	Flora Wakefield	Winston-Salem
1934	Hettie Reinhardt	Flora Wakefield	Fayetteville
1935	Ruth Council	Lucy Price	Charlotte
1936	Ruth Council	Lucy Price	Wilson
1937	Ruth Council	Lucy Price	Durham
1938	E. Irby Long (Mrs.)	Catherine C. Battie (Mrs.)	Asheville

APPENDIX C

NORTH CAROLINA BOARD OF NURSE EXAMINERS
1903-1938

1903
Marion H. Laurance (Mrs.),
president
Mary L. Wyche, secretary-
treasurer
Constance E. Pfohl
J. W. Long, M.D.
R. S. Primrose, M.D.

1904-1906
Constance E. Pfohl, president
Mary L. Wyche, secretary-
treasurer
Cleone E. Hobbs
J. W. Long, M.D.
R. S. Primrose, M.D.

1907-1908
Constance E. Pfohl, president
Mary L. Wyche, secretary-
treasurer
Anna Lee de Vane
J. E. Ashcraft, M.D.
John G. Blount, M.D.

1909-1911
Cleone E. Hobbs, president
Anne Ferguson, secretary-
treasurer
Maria P. Allen

C. A. Julian, M.D.
Oscar McMullin, M.D.

1912-1914
Ella MacNichols, president
Lois A. Toomer, secretary-
treasurer
Eugenia Henderson
J. W. Neal, M.D.
A. B. Croom, M.D.

1915-1916
Thompson Frazier, M.D.,
president
Lois A. Toomer, secretary-
treasurer
Maria P. Allen
Julia Lebby
Delia Dixon Carrol, M.D.
(deceased)

1917
Maria P. Allen, president
Lois A. Toomer, secretary-
treasurer
Julia Lebby
Delia Dixon Carrol, M.D.
(deceased)
Thompson Frazier, M. D.

1918

Maria P. Allen, president
Julia Lebby, secretary-treasurer
Lois A. Toomer
G. C. Battle, M.D. (resigned);
James Parrott, M.D., elected
July, 1918
Delia Dixon Carrol, M.D.
(deceased)

1919

Maria P. Allen, president
Julia Lebby, secretary-treasurer
Edith Redwine
C. F. Strosnider, M.D.
James M. Parrott, M.D.

1920

Lois A. Toomer, president
Effie E. Cain, secretary-treasurer
Edith Redwine
C. F. Strosnider, M.D.
James M. Parrott, M.D.

1921

Lois A. Toomer, president
Effie E. Cain, secretary-treasurer
Mary P. Laxton
C. F. Strosnider, M.D.
James M. Parrott, M.D.

1922

Lois A. Toomer, president
Dorothy Hayden (Mrs),
secretary-treasurer
Mary P. Laxton
James M. Parrott, M.D.
A. D. Stanton, M.D.

1923-1924

Mary P. Laxton, president
Dorothy Conyers (Mrs.),
secretary-treasurer

E. A. Kelley
James M. Parrott, M.D.
Oren Moore, M.D.

1925-1926

Mary P. Laxton, president
Dorothy Conyers (Mrs.),
secretary-treasurer
E. A. Kelley
R. Duval Jones, M.D.
Oren Moore, M.D.

1927

E. A. Kelley, president
Dorothy Conyers (Mrs.),
secretary-treasurer
Lula West
R. Duval Jones, M.D.
Oren Moore, M.D.

1928

E. A. Kelley, president
Dorothy Conyers (Mrs.),
secretary-treasurer
Lula West
R. W. Petrie, M.D.
Frank Sharpe, M.D.

1929

Lula West, president
Dorothy Conyers (Mrs.),
secretary-treasurer
Bessie M. Chapman
R. W. Petrie, M.D.
Frank Sharpe, M.D.

1930

Bessie M. Chapman, president
Dorothy Conyers (Mrs.),
secretary-treasurer
Josephine Kerr
R. W. Petrie, M.D.
Frank Sharpe, M.D.

1931

Bessie M. Chapman, president
Dorothy Conyers (Mrs.),
  secretary-treasurer
Josephine Kerr
D. A. Garrison, M.D.
C. H. Peete, M.D.

1932-1933

Bessie M. Chapman, president
Lula West, secretary-treasurer
Josephine Kerr
D. A. Garrison, M.D.
C. H. Peete, M.D.

1934

Bessie M. Chapman, president
Lula West, secretary-treasurer
Josephine Kerr
C. H. Peete, M.D.
B. C. Willis, M.D.

1935

Josephine Kerr, president
Bessie M. Chapman,
  secretary-treasurer
Hettie Reinhardt

C. H. Peete, M.D.
B. C. Willis, M. D.

1936

Josephine Kerr, president
Bessie Chapman,
  secretary-treasurer
Hettie Reinhardt
Marvin Scruggs, M.D.
H. A. Newell, M.D.

1937

Josephine Kerr, president
Bessie M. Chapman, secretary-
  treasurer
Hettie Reinhardt
Moir S. Martin, M.D.
H. A. Newell, M.D.

1938

Josephine Kerr, president
Bessie M. Chapman, secretary-
  treasurer
Martha C. Newman
Moir S. Martin, M.D.
H. A. Newell, M.D.

APPENDIX D

NORTH CAROLINA NURSES WHO SERVED IN THE WORLD WAR

Army Nurses*

†Abernathy, June Esther
Addor, Jeanne S.
†Aldridge, Johnsie M.
†Allen, Anna W.
†Allison, Rose
†Anderson, Lela E.
†Andler, Mary Morris
Armstrong, Vallie C.
†Arrington, Harriet L.
Arthur, Lucille E.
Ashby, Josie A.
†Ashton, Margaret V.
Atkins, Daisy R.
†Avent, Jessie E.
†Bailey, Edith L.
†Barker, Mary C.
Barringer, Frances A.
Baumberger, Lina
†Beam, Cora E.
†Benge, Mae F.
Benson, Laura Hutchins
Berg, Henrietta Van Den
Biggers, Blandina
Blackwelder, Estelle
†Blue, Jean F.
†Bodenheimer, Bess Blaine

Bowen, Alice M.
†Boyd, Lola Janet
†Branch, Mary Ione
†Britt, Lillian
Bryson, Margaret F.
†Burt, Katherine F.
†Butt, Hartley
†Casey, Alice Bertha
†Chalmers, Mary
†Chambers, Odessa
Chrisman, Luella
Christy, Julia B.
Clark, Laura Polly
†Clingman, Elizabeth C.
Coffield, Rena May
Coleman, Lucy G.
†Colson, Julia A.
†Compton, Clara M.
Cook, Lucille L.
†Corpening, Adah C.
†Crews, Grace K.
Crook, Annie M.
Crowell, Lillie H.
Crutchfield, Betty
†Dearman, Coral
Dent, Olga

* List from Adjutant General's Office, Washington, D. C.
† Nurses in service overseas.

Dick, Annie B.
†Doub, Laura Catherine
†Downey, Rosa A.
†Edwards, Bertha Lawrence
†Elliott, Maud V.
†Evans, Mary C.
†Ferguson, Rosalie
†Finch, Josephine
Fish, Ovah M.
Fisher, Faye
†Fly, Ella
Ford, Elizabeth A.
   (Mrs. Jack Shope)
†Fortune, Irma
†Fraley, Ruby
†Fredere, Clara R.
†Gallagher, Sadie Cecelia
Goforth, Mary Beall
Graham, Margaret J.
†Gray, Alice Shelton
Green, Annie M.
Greenfield, May
Grist, Mary Helen
Guy, Prudence Victoria
Hampton, Ruth
Hamrick, Mabel K.
†Harris, Ada Estelle
†Harris, Sara Myrtle
Hawley, Vannie May
†Hayden, Dorothy (Mrs.)
Hengeveld, Grace M.
†Henley, Maud L.
†Hill, Edna M.
†Hill, Elizabeth
†Hobbs, Cleone E.
†Hooten, Bessie E.
Hudson, Maud G.
Hunter, Johnnie B.
†Ikard, Ada Catherine
†Isley, Cora Laid

†Johnson, Gaye
Johnson, Grace B.
†Johnson, Hannah Al
†Johnson, John Ora
†Jones, Lucy A.
†Jones, Martha Elma
†Josey, Ethel M.
Kinsland, Daisy Eugenia
†Kirkpatrick, Minnie M.
Kensworthy, Helen
Kuykendall, Hallie L.
†Lambeth, Lula
Lea, Anna Katherine
†Leonard, Blanche Jettie
†Loman, Rachel M.
London, Lou E.
Long, Ethel
†Low, Sarah Elizabeth
†Lowry, Hattie Glendora
Lynch, Fleta A.
†MacKenzie, Ethel
†MacKenzie, Florence E.
May, Vivian Floranell
McBroom, Annie Lillian
McBroom, Edith Ellen
McCarley, Betty L.
McGhee, Estelle H.
†McIntosh, Montie
McKay, Ella C.
McKay, Hellen C.
†McNeill, Sue M.
†Memory, Fay
Miller, Ila Ethel
Miller, Stella
†Mills, Lois
Montgomery, Blanche A.
Moore, Elizabeth
Moore, Latta V.
†Moore, Sue Jane
†Morton, Emily

† Nurses in service overseas.

Moose, Annie L.
†Newman, Martha C.
†Niblock, Mable
†Nichols, Bert Carol
†O'Kelly, Manie
†Oates, Louise
†Osborn, Katherine
†Owen, Eufer
Parker, Annie L.
Patterson, Annie Washington
Patterson, Lula T.
Patton, Hazel N.
†Payne, Letitia
Penny, Frances Woodrow
‡Perkins, Etta Mae
†Petteway, Gertrude
Pettway, Stella
†Phifer, Pearl
†Pierce, Maud Estelle
†Potts, Mable
†Powell, Bessie D. (Mrs.)
†Range, Leah
†Reaves, Allie S.
Redding, Mary
†Reinhardt, Hettie
†Reinhardt, Louise
†‡Reveley, Annie Dade
†Richards, Elizabeth Catherine
Robbs, Mae
Robinson, Lelia J.
Robinson, Pauline
†Roddey, Harriet
†Rogers, Nora Rebecca
†Ruth, Clara Louise
Setzer, Maude B.
†Shackford, Mattie T.
†Shannon, Rosetta M.

Sigmon, Bertie May
Silver, Marie H.
Simpson, Nettie
Smith, Adele E.
†Smith, Elizabeth Herbert
Smith, Pearle
Sparks, Nola Ruth
†Staley, Minnie E.
†Stanford, Macie M.
Staton, Cora Jane
Stowe, Xanie
†Swearngan, Bess
Tate, Elizabeth
Tatum, A. Gertrude
†Taylor, Nora Louise
Thomas, Mary L.
†Tillingblast, Carolina Williams
†Timberlake, Mamie Louise
Toomer, Lois A.
†Trull, Lona E.
†Ulrick, Mamie
Utley, Minerva Ruffin
Vestal, Mozella
†Waters, Elizabeth
†Watts, Josephine
Weaver, L. Alberta
†Weaver, M. Pearl
Welch, Nora Amanda
†West, Lula
Whisenant, Eldy
†White, Martha Elizabeth
White, Martha Phylena
†Wicker, Ruth
†Williams, Eva
†Williams, Lottie E.
Wilkes, Maggie
†Yow, Annie

† Nurses in service overseas.
‡ Died in service.

Navy Nurses*

Anderson, Mary Jordan (Mrs.)
Aman, Lila M.
Campbell, Gertrude N.
Coleman, Maude
Collins, Helen Kate
DeLancy, Annie E.
Hamlin, Hazel D.
Harmon, Vera O.
Iseley, Myrtle
McClain, Helen

McLean, Lucy
Merritt, Annie Lee
Morgan, Mabel
Moss, Eva B.
Rogers, Bonnie May
Simmons, Mary Cordelia
Speas, Carolyn O.
Stockton, May E.
Thompson, Bertie A.

* List from Navy Department.

BIBLIOGRAPHY

American Red Cross Records.

Anderson, Mrs. John Huske (Lucy London), *North Carolina Women of the Confederacy*. Fayetteville, Cumberland Printing Co., 1926.

Clewell, John Henry, *History of Wachovia in North Carolina,* The Unitas Fratrum or Moravian Church in North Carolina during a century and a half. New York, Doubleday, Page & Co., 1902.

—— *Wachovia During the Revolution.*

Colonial Records of North Carolina. Edited by William L. Saunders. 10 vols. Raleigh, P. M. Hale, 1886-1890.

Consolidated Statutes of North Carolina. Annotated by A. C. McIntosh. Raleigh, Commercial Printing Co., 1919.

Draper, Lyman C., *King's Mountain and Its Heroes.* New York, Dauber & Pine Bookshops, Inc., 1929.

Ellet, Elizabeth F., *Women of the American Revolution.* 3 vols. New York, C. Scribner, 1851.

Files of North Carolina Newspapers.

Fries, Adelaide L. (ed.), *Records of the Moravians in North Carolina, 1758-1783.* 4 vols. Publications of the North Carolina Historical Commission. Raleigh, Edwards & Broughton, 1922-1930.

Hamilton, Joseph Grégoire deRoulhac, *History of North Carolina Since 1860.*

—— *Reconstruction in North Carolina.* New York, Longmans, Green & Co., 1914.

McMasters, John Bach, *A History of the People of the United States During Lincoln's Administration.* New York and London, D. Appleton & Co., 1927.

Marshall, Helen E., *Dorothea Dix, Forgotten Samaritan.* Chapel Hill, The University of North Carolina Press, 1937.

Minutes of the North Carolina State Nurses' Association, 1902-1936.

North Carolina Booklet. 23 vols. Raleigh, North Carolina Society, Daughters of the American Revolution, 1901-1923.

North Carolina State Records, Vols. IV, XV.

Nutting, Mary Adelaide, and Dock, Lavinia L., *A History of Nursing.* 2 vols. New York and London, G. P. Putnam's Sons, 1907.

Personal Narratives.

Public Laws of North Carolina, 1903, 1907, 1917, 1919, 1925, 1931, 1933.

Rhodes, James Ford, *History of the Civil War 1861-1865.* New York, The Macmillan Company, 1917.

Simkins, Francis Butler, and Patton, James Welch, *The Women of the Confederacy.* Richmond and New York, Garrett & Massie, Inc., 1936.

Southern Hospital, Vol. III, 1935; Vol. IV, 1936; Vol. V, No. 5, 1937.

Wheeler, John H., *Historical Sketches of North Carolina, from 1584 to 1851.* Compiled from original records, official documents and traditional statements. Philadelphia, Lippincott, Grambo & Co., 1851.

INDEX

ADAMS, Dr. R. M., 43
Anderson, Dr. Albert, 29, 45
Anderson, Dr. T. E., 43
Andrews, Fannie V., 39
Archer, Dr. I. J., 111
Asheville Mission Hospital, 38-39

BAKER, Bessie, 49, 79, 83
Barbee, Mrs. C. B., 34, 125
Batterham, Mary Rose, 52-53, 68, 69, 84
Battle, Dr. K. P., Jr., 31, 35
Battle, Judge W. H., 32
Beam, Cora E., 118
Beasley, Mrs., 15
Bell, Celeste, 74
Bell, Martha McFarlane, 13
Berry, Margaret, 22
Bitting, Mrs. J. A., 40
Blair, Dr. Elizabeth, 50
Board of Nurse Examiners, 72, 74, 90, 112; members of, 138-40
Bodie, Marion, 127
Bonn, Dr. Jacob, 7, 8
Bride, Mary, 46
Broadfoot, Carrie E., 129-31
Brown, Jane, 82
Browne, Dr., 11
Buie, Miss M. A., 18
Bunn, J. W., 34
Burgess, Marie L., 128
Burnett, Dr. F. F., 129
Buxton, Fannie, 51, 52
Buxton, Mrs. James G., 40

CAIN, Lucille, 85
Carlton, Dr. R. S., 123
Carrington, Dr. G. L., 88
Carter, Helen P., 129
Case, Ella, 69
Chalmers, Daisy D., 87

Chapman, Bessie, 94
City Hospital of Wilmington, 35-36
City Memorial Hospital, 40-43
Clark, Rev. W. M., 31
Clay, Ethel, 44
Clingman, Elizabeth, 25, 80
Cochran, Mrs. Eva S., 45
Coffin, Jennie, 31
Cohen, Ida Reid, 82
Collins, Geneva S., 130
Community Hospital, 129
Conyers, Dorothy (Mrs.), 25, 48, 62, 80
Cooper, Dr. George M., 117-18
Corker, Lottie C., 35, 83
Cotchett, Lossie deRosset, 64
Council, Ruth, 83, 84
Courts, Mollie, 22
Crews, Laura, 42
Crowson, Nannie Lou, 55-56, 69
Currie, Nola, 89

DAVIS, Nell, 83
Delano, Jane A., 23, 79
Denmark, Mrs. Walter, 89
DeRosset, Mrs. Armand, 19
Dickson, Mrs. Clyde, 122
Dimm, Louise, 38
Districts, organization of, 85-86
Dix, Dorothea Lynde, 27
Dix Hill, 28
Dobbin, James C., 27
Dorothea Dix School of Nursing, 29
Duke, J. B., 48
Duke University School of Nursing, 48-49
Dunn, Birdie, 54-55, 112, 115, 118
Dunnwyche, 54, 59, 62, 111 ff.

EAST, Louise P., 89
Educational Directors, 90

Ehrenfield, Rose M., 84
Elliott, Mrs. Sarah E., 19-20
Ericson, Oliva, 85

Faires, Lillian, 83
Farley, Marie, 83, 84
Farmer, Nina Lewis, 64-65
Ferguson, Anne, 22, 43, 58-59, 69
Fisher, Dr. Edward C., 28
Fisher, Newton, 88
Fogle, Mary Anne, 40
Foreman, Mildred, 83
Freeman, Lucia, 84

Gilliland, Selena, 42
Goodman, Katherine, 85
Good Samaritan Hospital, 126
Gordon, Ruby, 25
Graham, Margaret J., 80
Gray, Mrs. James A., Sr., 40
Groves, Annie, 127, 129
Guffy, Mrs. H. P., 118

Hall, Della J., 22
Hall, Mrs. J. O., 40
Hall, Myrtle R., 29
Hanner, Miss, 48
Hardister, Sallie, 80
Harper, Mrs. John, 20
Hauser, Blanche, 65
Hawkins, Myrtle, 74
Hay, Helen S., 81
Hayden, Dr. Catherine P., 128
Hayden, Dorothy. *See* Conyers, Dorothy
Hayes, Florence, 37
Health work, city and county, 120-25;
    in schools, 118, 123-24
Heinzerling, Edna L., 83
Heller, M. Lilly, 37
Henderson, L. Eugenia, 60-61
Henderson, Miss Z. B., 69
Hendrix, Moselle, 118
Hengeveld, Grace, 80
Highsmith, Dr. J. F., Sr., 45, 88
Highsmith Hospital, 45-46
Hill, Dr. J. W., 43
Hill, Rosa G., 35
Hines, Dr. Peter E., 31, 35

Hobbs, Cleone E., 25, 56-57, 79, 80,
    118
Holman, Lydia, 59-60
Horry, Mary, 122
Hospitals. *See name of individual hospital*
House, Abbey Horne, 18
Howland, Elizabeth, 19
Hudson, Dr. C. C., 123

Idol, Lelia M., 82
Industrial Nurse Section, State Nurses'
    Association, 89
Infant hygiene, 119
In Memoriam, 132-34
Insanity, treatment of, 27

James Walker Memorial Hospital,
    36-38
Johnson, Agnes B., 46
Johnson, Lessie, 29
Johnson, Dr. N. M., 123
Jones, Stella, 46
Josey, Ethel, 25

Kalberlahn, Dr. H. Martin, 5,
    6, 7
Kay, Dr. John, 129
Kelley, Essie Alma (E. A.), 46, 63-64,
    76, 83, 89, 115
Kelly, Betty, 48
Kelly, Sibbie, 80
Kennedy, Mrs. C. C., 15
Kestler, Ethel, 64
Kings' Daughters Hospital, 39-40
Kinyoun, Dr. J. J., 123
Knox, Dr. A. W., 31, 35
Kuykendall, Hallie, 80
Kyle, Annie K., 19

Lambe, Blanche, 84
Lane, Dr. W. Walter, 36
Large, Dr. H. J., 88
Latta, Edward D., 39
Latta, Julia A., 129
Laurance, Mrs. Marion H., 69, 72, 74,
    95
Lawrison, Amelia, 121
Laxton, Mary P., 57-58, 75, 77, 83

League of Nursing Education, 75-79
Lebby, Julia, 81
Legislation for Nurses, 95 ff.
Lehey, Frances, 48
LeMay, Thomas J., 32
Leonard Hospital, 127
Lester, Dr. Harry L., 88
Lewis, Dr. Richard H., 31, 117
Lincoln Hospital, 129
Litchford, James, 32
Little, Dr. Thomas R., 37
Livingston, Kate, 118
Lofton, Mary, 83
Long, Dr. Henry F., 43
Long, Hortense, 43
Long, Dr. John Wesley, 23, 72
Long's Hospital, 43-44, 59
Lowe, Dr. Charles E., 124
Lowry, Hattie, 24, 74, 79, 80, 85

McCOMBS, Mrs. J. B., 22
McDuffie, Catherine, 87
McGee, Dr. James W., 34
McKay, Virginia, 39, 77, 88
McKee, Dr. James, 29, 31, 35
McLean, Jessie, 83
McLester, Maggie, 31
McNeil, Effie E., 30
McNeil, Mattie S., 24, 64
MacNichols, Caroline, 30
MacNichols, Ella H., 75, 79, 81
McPhaul, Dr. W. A., 124
MacRae, Evelina, 51
Manguin, Miss, 48
Mason, Louise, 83
May, Mary Bell, 50
Maynard, Betty, 48
Mercy Hospital, 46-48
Military nursing, 9-25. See also Nurses, in World War
Mimms, Nora P., 35
Missionaries, nurses as, 64-65
Moore, Dr. C. E., 45
Moore, Mary E., 83
Moore, Mattie, 85
Moore, Naomi, 83
Moravians, 5 ff.
Mordecai, Elizabeth, 35

Morris, Annie, 45
Morris, Effie, 45
Mosley, Laura, 65
Mott, Susan, 30
Munds, Columbia, 61-62, 83, 84, 88, 115, 124
Muse, Gilbert, 77
Myers, Katherine, 84

NEGRO hospitals, 126-30
Negro nurses, 126 ff.; associations of, 126, 130-31
Newsome, Ella K., 18
Nurses, in World War, army, 141-43; navy, 144. See also missionaries
Nurses, organizations of, 66-89
Nurses' Relief Fund, 54, 111, 115
Nursing, in public schools. See Health work
Nursing Schools, 26-50

OFFICE Nurse Section, State Nurses' Association, 89
Oldham, Mary, 85
Oldham, Minnie, 45
Orr, Adeline, 53

PALMER, Eva, 35
Parrot, Dr. J. M., 87
Peace, William, 32
Perkins, Etta Mae, 25
Perry, Florence M., 80
Petteway, Gertrude, 80
Pettigrew, Mrs. M. L., 15
Pettway, Stella, 80
Pfohl, Constance E., 55, 72, 74, 79, 80, 81
Pickard, Emily J., 122
Pioneers, in nursing, 51 ff.
Powers, Alice A., 30
Powers, Percy, 80, 121, 123
Presbyterian Hospital, 50
Primrose, Dr. R. S., 72
Private Duty Section, State Nurses' Association, 85
Professional registries, 83-84
Public health, 60, 120, 122; nursing, 116 ff., 125. See also Health work

Public Health Section, State Nurses' Association, 84
Purnell, Elizabeth, 35

Raulston, Mrs. Lewis, 123
Ray, Flora, 118
Red Cross Nursing Committee, 55, 79
Red Cross Nursing Service, 79-83
Redwine, Edith M., 74, 76, 91
Registration, for nurses, 95 ff.
Reinhardt, Hettie, 24, 80, 87
Reinhardt, Louise, 24
Reveley, Annie Dade, 25
Rex, John, 31
Rex Hospital, 31-34
Rex Hospital School for Nurses, 34-35
Reynolds, Mrs. G. E., 124
Reynolds, R. J., 42-43
Reynolds, Mrs. R. J., 43
Rich, Rev. E. R., 31
Richardson, Mrs. L., 130
Richardson Memorial Hospital, 130
Robertson, Myrtle F., 122
Robinson, Alberta, 37
Robinson, Mary E., 46
Rogers, Mrs. J. M., 41
Ross, Clara, 83, 84, 124
Royal, Dr. B. F., 88
Royster, Dr. Hubert, 128

St. Agnes Hospital, 127-29
St. John's Guild, 31
St. John's Hospital, 31, 32
St. Leo's Hospital, 48
St. Peter's Hospital, 29-31
Sanders, Mary F., 20
Scarlette, Ruby F., 131
Schools of Nursing. See Nursing Schools
Schultz, Anna D., 22
Shaffner, Mrs. J. F., 41
Sharp, Lucy Abbey, 22
Shelton, Louise, 89
Shore, Mrs. E. D., 34
Shore, Ethel, 83
Sloan, Mary, 118
Slocumb, Captain Ezekiel, 12
Slocumb, Mary, 12-13
Smith, Ella Price, 42
Smith, Richard, 32

Smith, Sterling, 43
Solomon, Beatrice, 83
Spach, Mollie E., 42, 53-54
Spenser, Elizabeth, 39
Squires, Beulah, 46
Stafford, Blanche, 62, 82, 83, 85
Standardization Board, 86-88
State Board of Health, 116 ff.
State Educational Directors, 90-94
State Hospital for the Insane, 27-29
State Nurses' Association, 66-72; charter members of, 135; past presidents and secretaries of, 136-37
State Relief Fund, 115
State Sanatorium, Negro division of, 129
Sternberger, Mrs. E., 130
Stinson, Julia, 74
Strong, Dr. C. M., 87
Strudwick, Dr. Edmund, 28
Sturgeon, Annie, 68, 69

Taylor, Salome, 129
Thomas, Mamie, 65, 80
Thomas, Nora, 45
Thomas, Dr. W. N., 88
Thompson, Ida, 74
Tilly, Lillian, 89
Toomer, Lois A., 90
Torrence, Estelle, 85
Trist, Mary H., 75
Tucker, Sadie, 33
Turner, Mrs. Kerenhappuck, 12
Tuttle, Ella, 22
Twin-City Hospital, 41, 42

Vane, Anne Lee de, 56, 69
Vogler, Maria, 40

Wakefield, Flora, 125
Walker, James, 36-37
Walker Memorial Hospital. See James Walker Memorial Hospital
Waller, Dr. C. E., 125
Watson, Ellen S., 42
Watts, George W., 44
Watts Hospital, 44-45
Wesson, Laura, 18-19
West, Kathleen, 29

West, Lula, 87, 93
Wheeler, Edna H., 128
Whittington, Dr. J. B., 87, 88
Wilkes, Mrs. John, 29
Williams, Hazel C., 31, 83
Williamson, Dr. Hugh, 9, 10
Williamson, W. H., 33
Willis, Dr. B. C., 87
Wilmington City Hospital. *See* City
    Hospital of Wilmington
Wilson Sanatorium, 45
Wood, Dr. Hugh F., 116-17

Worral, Mrs. Frances, 129
Wortham, Effie, 129
Wren, Betty, 20
Wren, Mrs. Mary, 20
Wright, Martha T., 124
Wright, W. B., 34
Wyche, Mary Lewis, 32, 34, 35, 44,
    66, 67, 68, 69, 72, 75, 79, 112

Y ANCEY, Jane Christmas, 51, 52
Yorke, Mrs. Mary L., 65